DEDICATION

T o the founders, staff, caregivers and patients of the George G. Glenner Alzheimer's Family Center. They are a wonderful, dedicated group doing a very difficult task in the best possible way.

ACKNOWLEDGMENTS

I would like to extend special thanks to my sister, Barbara, for her encouragement and her seemingly endless assistance with the computer; to my brother-in-law, Harley, for his encouragement; to my sister, Jean, and her husband, Art, for their optimism; and to Debra Lee Baldwin, for her confidence and positive attitude. To my dear friend, Pat Gay, who shared her thoughts with me. And, finally, to all the patients and caregivers whose thoughts, problems and feelings are encompassed in this book.

I also feel that I had my dear parents, Tom and Catherine Higgins and my husband, Jerry, smiling down at me from Heaven while I was writing these few pages.

CONTENTS

DISCLAIMER

I have fictionalized names and case histories used as examples throughout this book. Any resemblance of persons or places mentioned in the book to actual persons or places is purely coincidental.

I do not claim to be an expert in the field of Alzheimer's disease care, but rather a person who has experience in caring for the ill.

My intent is to offer suggestions that should help caregivers and their loved ones have happier, more peaceful lives. It helps to know you are not the only one with a problem, and that there is someone who truly understands.

Your personal physician should be the decision maker when it comes to the medical care your loved one receives.

Eileen Higgins Driscoll
R.N.(retired)

FOREWORD

I hope, by writing this book, I am able to lighten your burden.

Alzheimer's disease is a family tragedy. It is catastrophic for the patient and for those around him. It is a most difficult illnesses to understand because you can't see it; yet, you witness its devastating effects.

Families often are overwhelmed by the ravages of Alzheimer's disease, which affects not only the patient but all significant others. The information within these pages is intended to help make the lives of those affected by Alzheimer's disease easier, in spite of the terrible situation they deal with daily.

The book is written for people who are not in the medical profession. I have attempted to simplify as much as possible and have stayed away from medical terminology, making the content as conversational as possible.

The thoughts, observations and opinions throughout are mine, accumulated over years of caretaking for family, friends and patients.

I do not deal with cause, effect or treatment of Alzheimer's disease from a primarily medical point of view. Rather, it is my intent to deal with the results of the disease from the caregiver's point of view, in order to assist in the daily care of the patient.

My heart goes out to anyone caught in the web of Alzheimer's disease. If what I have written helps you even a little bit, then this book is successful.

Eileen Higgins Driscoll
R.N.(retired)

PREFACE

Alzheimer's Disease presents a true test of human resources for the burdened family caregiver. This is a caregiver's handbook written with a loving voice by a professional caregiver.

Inevitably the best ideas are often the simplest, and the most obvious. However, it is difficult to be realistic in coping strategies when fatigue and frustration overcome the best of intentions.

This "Sharing the Caring" experiences by Eileen Driscoll is her tender loving voice reaching out to help others in providing a "Celebration of Life" for the Alzheimer's patient.

Joy Glenner
Executive Director
Co-founder

The George G. Glenner
Alzheimer's Family Center's Inc.
San Diego, California

Chapter One

Attitude is Everything

What do you mean, you got lost on the way home?"

Before something big (like forgetting the way home) happens, most caregivers have noticed more subtle signs of Alzheimer's disease. Caregivers often let these go by as mistakes anyone might make.

For example, you may have observed "filling in" that the patient makes something up rather than admit he or she forgot. In the early stages of the disease, patients often are very aware of their forgetfulness and other errors, and are busy covering up those errors. At the same time, they are ashamed and upset with their own actions.

One lady, whom I'll call Amanda, told me the way her mother would take telephone messages. Once she told Amanda her husband had called, and that he wanted to meet her at Main and Fifth streets at five o'clock. Amanda went and waited. Her husband never came, and she returned home. After consulting her husband, Amanda discovered he had said a different street and time. After several other wrong messages, they realized there was something wrong with Mother. A doctor confirmed their concerns.

Caregivers often deny that anything is wrong with their loved ones. It is difficult to believe a person you've counted on as a pillar of strength is not as strong as he or she once was, and, as a matter of fact, is quite vulnerable.

What are you going to do? Once you acknowledge something is amiss, it is important to have a doctor establish a diagnosis. There are many diseases that mimic Alzheimer's. Some of them are very easily treated, and if this is the case, your troubles and worries are behind you.

However, if Alzheimer's disease is the diagnosis, don't be discouraged; a great deal of research is being done and treatment should be available in the near future.

When you really are feeling your worst and don't know what to do, I have a suggestion that may, at first, sound ridiculous. Try a hug. Yes, just put your arms around the sick one and hug. You will both feel better. It is surprising how far a little love can go, and what it can accomplish. Not only will you both feel better, this will help you to maintain your priority: the best care for the patient. Remember, the sick one is confused, upset and unable to express feelings, but love and touch are basic needs and we all respond to them.

Understanding the disease

Alzheimer's does not respect intelligence, education, walk of life, money, or any of the other amenities we know in this world. It is a thief in the night that robs the patient of his or her very self, a little at a time.

The five stages listed in this chapter are the best way I can describe the progress of the disease. Some people might prefer to call them five aspects. There is no clear cut beginning or end to a stage, and the sick person can go back and forth from one stage to the other several times in one day.

Much has been researched, written and said about Alzheimer's disease, and there is still much more to be discovered. The brain is a wonderful organ and is very complex. Therefore, it is difficult to know why it is not functioning properly.

In order for you to understand what is happening in the brain of an Alzheimer's patient, let me share a particularly appropriate metaphor with you.

George G. Glenner, MD, president, founder and medical director of the Alzheimer's Family Center in San Diego, describes the progression of Alzheimer's disease this way:

Imagine a small light for every function of the brain. These lights are fed by electricity. Now imagine that the electricity to one light is cut off. That light will go out but the difference is difficult to notice because all the other lights are still on. This is the very beginning of Alzheimer's disease.

Now imagine that the voltage to all the lights has lessened. The lights are still on but they are not as bright as they once were. This is the slow progression noticeable in Alzheimer's disease. Then, one by one, ever so slowly, the electricity to one light at a time is cut off. Some of the lights are still on but they are very dim; this is further progression of the disease.

The lights never all go out but are left with too little light to be effective. They need the assistance of another light to function. As the caregiver, YOU are this other light.

Stages of the disease

Your doctor will advise you, on an individual basis, concerning the progression of Alzheimer's disease. Below is an outline of how I have observed the disease and its stages. Some patients go from one stage to another very rapidly; others may skip a stage or stay in one for a long time; and, often, stages may overlap.

Stage One: Aware. The patient is aware of his or her forgetfulness. He or she is embarrassed, angry and denies errors; blames others; and "fills in" by fabricating forgotten information. The patient is aware of making errors yet is unable to understand why. Caregivers should remember it is very important to give reassurance at this stage, and during the next.

Stage Two: Acceptance. The patient accepts the diagnosis of Alzheimer's disease and its ramifications. He or she has damage in one area of the brain; other areas function in an apparently normal manner. Caregivers should keep in mind that some patients develop insight when they first become ill. They understand and accept the diagnosis, and, because they know the bleak future that awaits them, the knowledge can be very painful for them.

Stage Three: Unaware. As the disease progresses the results of brain damage become more apparent. The patient becomes unaware of his or her problems and is less able to prevent, cope or otherwise hide problem behaviors. Patients may not recognize their caregivers or their own homes. Understandably, this is a very difficult bridge for all concerned to cross.

Stage Four: Partial Care. At this point, the patient has trouble dressing and bathing himself. The patient may "forget" to go to the bathroom until it is too late. You may notice more bizarre behavior for which the patient is not responsible; at this point he has no control. Caregivers may have to help with feeding.

Stage Five: Full Care. You, as caregiver, assume total responsibility for the patient; whatever is needed for his or her comfort and well being is now your job. Just like caring for an infant, you must feed, dress, diaper and do all other "activities of daily living" to assist the patient.

The five stages listed above will be discussed in greater detail in later chapters. You will learn how to recognize them, how to deal with them, and how understand each from a very different viewpoint: the patient's. Whenever appropriate, I also have included illustrations of stages and symptoms from (fictionalized) case histories.

Maintain a positive attitude

You must remember: ONCE Alzheimer's disease IS DIAGNOSED, THE PATIENT IS EXCUSED ONE HUNDRED PERCENT OF THE TIME. If you start with this premise you will make your life and the patient's life much easier and happier.

Keep your sense of humor. If something happens that doesn't really matter, learn to say, "So what?" Rather than fussing over something unimportant, let it go.

You may have to establish a whole new set of priorities due to this dramatic change in your life. Whether you like it or not, you have no choice but to deal with it.

If you expect nothing positive from the patient, anything you do receive from him or her is a bonus for you. It may take a while to adjust your line of thinking in this vein, but I assure you, if you do so, your days will be happier and you will be less frustrated.

People understand a broken arm because they can see it, but few understand a broken brain. Alzheimer's disease makes the patient do "wrong things" that remain inexplicable.

It also helps to keep in mind that the sick person is your loved one, and he has earned a special place through his own giving of himself to you. He has been a good parent (or spouse, or friend). Now it is your turn.

You also should realize you do have a choice: You don't have to do the care personally. There are alternatives. If you are caring for your loved one, you are doing so because you have chosen to do so.

Never allow anyone to make you feel ashamed of your sick loved one. Some people are rude or ignorant and may make remarks that make you feel bad. Keep in mind that no one ever wants to get Alzheimer's disease. Moreover, no one has a guarantee that it will never happen to him or her.

Throughout the book, we will discuss the reactions and feelings caregivers typically experience, and how to deal with these in a positive, productive manner.

Medical needs, behavior changes

There may be other illnesses present in a patient with Alzheimer's disease. The patient's medical doctor will address these problems and prescribe for them. Frequently a patient will have poor sight or hearing, which compounds the communication problem between caregiver and patient. Often glasses and hearing aids, though very necessary, are other nuisances to contend with.

Behavior changes may indicate a need for sedatives or stimulants. Again, the doctor will be able to assess these needs and prescribe for them. Unfortunately, patients may vacillate from one extreme to the other over the course of an hour or so, which makes the caregiver's job more difficult.

If your patient is unable or unwilling to swallow a pill, some medications come in liquid form and can be administered with a little applesauce, ice cream or pudding. If there is no liquid form of the medicine, most pills can be crushed and mixed with soft foods. Be sure to check with your pharmacist first, however. There are some medications that should not be crushed or opened.

The most stressful and potentially dangerous behavior change is the catastrophic reaction. This is something you, as caregiver, will want to try to avoid. These escalating moods of agitation occur for reasons that are often not clearly understood, because they start in a mind disturbed by a disease which is a form of dementia.

When you realize the patient's mood is escalating in a direction that is unfavorable, there are things you can do (apart from medication) to try to stop it in its early stages. We will discuss this in detail in Chapter Four.

Dealing with a catastrophic reaction is one of the most difficult challenges for the caregiver. It is particularly difficult, at this time, to remember the patient is NOT RESPONSIBLE AND IS ONE HUNDRED PERCENT EXCUSED.

You will find yourself at wit's end, saying to yourself, "What should I do?" Well, just do your best. You can do no more than that, and what you are doing is wonderful: You are taking care of a loved one as best you can.

We all decide what is important in life and then pattern our lives accordingly. You have decided that the care of your loved one is the important thing to do, now, at this time of your life.

Chapter Two
Know Your Limitations

A competent physician has diagnosed your loved one as having Alzheimer's disease. Chances are, he or she is not too sick at this time. Even though the patient is making mistakes, there haven't been any terribly bad ones. Your confidence in yourself allows you to believe, "Oh, I'll manage just fine even though it will be a little troublesome."

Unfortunately, this is not true. You are going to need help, and lots of it, before you are finished. Now is the time to lay your plans on the table.

I have seen caregivers defer seeking help or a support system until their situations reached a point where everything was in turmoil, both for patient and caregiver. In one situation, the caregiver lost self-control and was hysterical.

This unfortunate occurrence can be avoided with some good concrete planning, during which you anticipate the crisis situation ahead.

You have to keep in mind, when doing your planning, that everyone has a different capacity, both emotional and physical. This has to be considered carefully, early on. Just because a certain person or family was able to care for a loved one does not mean that everyone is capable of doing the same thing.

We have established two important facts:

-- The patient is very ill and will need long term care, which will become increasingly difficult.

-- It is unlikely you will be able to do all of the care by yourself.

In order to take the best possible care of the patient, the caregiver must maintain his or her physical and mental health. In other words: You must take care of the caregiver. How can you go about doing this?

Care for the caregiver

It is imperative that the caregiver have a complete medical check-up, now, to be sure he or she is physically able to care for the patient. You must know this in the beginning, because all your plans will rest squarely on the caregiver's shoulders.

Keep in mind, as time goes by and the patient's disease progresses, caregiving will become more and more physically difficult for the caregiver. If he or she is not well it would be wise to make plans for the patient to be placed outside the home, or for another person to be in the home daily to share the work.

I realize this is a decision no one wants to make, but if you don't make it now, when you have time to plan ahead, it will have to be made in haste when a crisis presents itself and you may have to take what is quickly available, rather than being able to choose carefully.

Consider, too, the mental health of the caregiver. The patient will need a stable environment, and the caregiver must supply that stability. It is easy to say, "Oh, I'm physically well and want to care for this person," but you must look to the future. The caregiver will need a release valve for the stress that is bound to accumulate. Again, planning for that should be done, now, in the early stages of the disease.

Family involvement

Sometimes a primary caregiver, patient and family live in the same household. If this is the situation, all members of the family should sit down and work out a plan together. If one member of the family is hesitant about providing care, that person should be excused rather than forced to contribute. If there will be constant upset in the household about the degree and kind of care given to the patient, it is better to place the patient in long term care, outside the home. This is preferable to having family members in a constant state of disagreement. They must work together in harmony.

There are many things we don't know about Alzheimer's disease, but we do know that the lifestyle of the patient and his or her loved ones will be dramatically changed by the illness. The family must deal with this fact, one way or another.

As I stated earlier, we all decide what is important in our lives and how we will deal with situations. We often don't choose circumstances that come our way, but we must deal with them, whether we like them or not. I believe God has His plans and sometimes it is not for us to understand why things happen.

It is important that the caregiver and all others concerned have an understanding of Alzheimer's disease in order to give proper care to the patient, and to help themselves do the care properly. Hopefully, this book will be helpful, but it would be good to read as much literature on the subject as possible. The goal is to better understand what is happening to your loved one.

I haven't told you many positive things since the beginning of this book. It might be helpful to mention now that there is great satisfaction in caregiving if it is done with the right attitude. I have been a caregiver all my life and I doubt any other career would have given me more satisfaction.

Of course, we are all different individuals, and not all of us are suited for caregiving. Those who are not should place their efforts elsewhere, perhaps overseeing the care of the loved one. Caregiving with the wrong attitude will lead to disaster, both for patient and caregiver.

You may recall I emphasized earlier that an Alzheimer's patient's behavior must be excused one hundred percent of the time. When a person is born the brain grows and develops daily. When a person has Alzheimer's disease the brain function deteriorates daily. Neither the newborn nor the Alzheimer's patient has any control over the degree of brain material available to him.

Love is essential to successful caregiving.

Join a support group

An Alzheimer's family support group has many things to offer which you may desperately need. It can give you an opportunity to share your problem, which will make it easier to bear. You will feel comforted, knowing you are not alone in your struggle. There are others who completely understand what you are going through, and who can empathize.

Sometimes you and members of your support group will shed a few tears together. This can be wonderful for all concerned. It is a safe way to release pent-up emotions you must keep under control day after day.

You will meet dependable people who understand your situation, who are knowledgeable, and who are only a phone call away. This can be invaluable if there is an emergency and you need help with hands-on care.

The support group will also offer you up-to-date information on work being done in the medical field to combat Alzheimer's disease. You also will learn ideas that will assist you in the care of your particular patient, and find out how to access professional help in your area as needed.

Respite care by professionals

There will come a point when friends and family members cannot provide enough, or adequate, respite care to relieve the overworked caregiver.

If there is an Alzheimer's day care center in your area, you will want to visit it and see if the patients are well cared for. If so, this can be an ideal source of respite. The cost is usually based on a sliding scale, so that it is affordable to all.

The patient can stay at the day care center for one or more days a week. This allows the caregiver a chance to rest or work without interruption, while the loved one is well cared for.

Your loved one must be cared for by people who understand the ravages of the illness, what it does to the brain, and the dementia that results from it. They also should be trained to handle any emergencies that might occur. Ask members of your support group if they are satisfied with the day care facility. Make sure the day care employees are professionally trained, and specialize in the care of Alzheimer's disease patients.

Introduce your loved one to day care slowly. A healthy mind has a lot of adjusting to do in a new environment. How much more adjusting does a sick mind have to do in a new environment? Your loved one has to understand he is going to a safe place with friendly people.

If you will be needing respite care for overnight or longer, there are facilities that will care for your loved one on a temporary basis. We will discuss these in Chapter Nine: Placement Outside the Home.

Love, but be objective

As an effective caregiver, you will try to:

-- Look at the positive side of what you are dealing with.

-- Realize you do have alternatives, even though you have made the choice to care for your loved one at home. You are doing this because you have decided this is what you WANT to do.

-- Do not allow yourself to feel like a martyr (which will depress you so much you will not be able to do the job objectively).

-- Anticipate, and find, great satisfaction in caring for your loved one. You see this satisfaction as a bonus you receive.

-- Also keep in mind that you need a respite frequently. You realize no one should undertake the job of full care without knowing in advance there will be opportunities to relax and have fun.

All this, of course, is easier said than done. The key to accomplishing it is to remain objective and loving at the same time. This might sound contradictory, but it really isn't. It is a skill, and it can be learned. I developed it in my early years as a student in a most unusual way.

Let me tell you how I learned, and how I manage. (I also encourage you to speak with others who have been, or are, successful caregivers. Put our ideas together, and you will likely discover the method that works best for you.)

When I was a nursing student in the late '40s, before tranquilizers were available, I affiliated for three months in a mental hospital. I arrived there with a very positive attitude.

I came from a sheltered childhood, and had no idea that such people existed. I was exposed to patients in manic stages, who were hallucinating and screaming, and who had no touch with reality. I saw people placed in straight jackets and canvas sheets, and I saw them tied to their beds. Often they were yelling as loud as they were able.

As you might imagine, the experience of watching all of this, without adequate preparation, caused me to run outside the hospital. Fortunately, a doctor on staff happened by and saw me laughing and crying and talking to myself. He realized I was hysterical and slapped my face until I stopped.

Over a cup of coffee, he explained the necessity for me to learn to be objective and loving at the same time. "You have to learn to detach yourself from the patient and look at the job to be done," he explained. "While you are doing this you have to tell yourself you are going to do the job in the kindest and most gentle way possible."

"And when you leave, you have to develop an imaginary window shade you pull down behind you, so that you can temporarily dismiss what you have been doing. While someone else is looking after the patient, you do not think about what is going on, and concern yourself only with what you are doing at the present. And, hopefully, what you are doing is something pleasant for you."

I have carried my shade with me for almost 50 years, and I put it up and down when needed. It works for me, and you must find a similar method that also works for you.

Chapter Three
Stage One: Aware

I suspect, when the illness first starts, even the patient is unaware that something is not quite right. We all forget a word or an appointment now and then and it means nothing except we merely forgot. Maybe we were over-loaded. (That's the excuse I always use when I forget something.) We squeeze too many activities into a short span of time, and something has to give.

The difference between this normal forgetfulness and Alzheimer's disease is that, after a while, the loved one realizes he is making too many mistakes and forgetting too many things. He or she knows something is amiss but does not yet know what is wrong.

Soon the patient starts to make an effort to cover his errors. He may be able to do this adequately for a while, but as the illness progresses, the cover-ups become less efficient.

Other people start to notice the errors. In the beginning, the errors are so subtle they easily go unnoticed. Sometimes the family members are the last to notice because they see the loved one daily and become used to the changes slowly. And at other times family members notice yet ignore the odd behavior because they don't want to admit, even to themselves, that something is wrong.

What do you think is happening to the patient's self-assurance while this is going on? He (or she) is becoming very upset, frightened and ashamed, and is unwilling to tell anyone what is happening. He worries about his job if he has one. He is concerned about what he can do to stop this terrible thing that is happening to him. He is afraid to tell anyone what is going on and won't even tell his family. Wouldn't that be an alarming situation to find yourself in?

Stage One symptoms

Here's a list of behaviors that begin early in the disease:

-- Difficulty in telling a story completely.

-- Difficulty in understanding a story or a joke.

-- Difficulty in telling a story correctly.

-- Loss of a train of thought in the middle of a sentence.

-- Misuse of a word.

-- Substituting one word for another.

-- Losing track of money or check book balances.

-- Misplacing belongings or losing them.

-- Forgetfulness (more than normal).

-- Inappropriate conversation.

-- Confusion during meals.

-- Wrong response to something said to him.

-- Failure to recognize a familiar person or place.

-- Confusion in unfamiliar situations.

-- Confusion in familiar situations.

-- Changes in manner of dress (unmatched clothing, no jacket when it is cold, etc.)

-- Inability to find something when it is in its proper place.

-- Taking longer that normal to complete a task.

-- Inability to complete a task.

-- Changes in sleep pattern.

-- Poor judgment in decision making.

-- Unable to make a decision.

-- Small mishaps with car (denting fender on way into garage, forgetting where car is parked).

-- Accidents with car.

-- Getting lost in car in familiar surroundings.

-- Getting lost while walking in familiar surroundings.

-- Unable to follow simple directions.

-- Inappropriate mood changes.

-- Flaccid facial appearance.

-- Answers yes or no instead of discussing something when a question is put to him or her (can't remember the answer).

-- Avoiding people outside the home.

-- Sleeping more than usual.

-- Withdrawing from activities.

-- Wide mood swings.

-- Poor coordination or balance.

-- Change in appetite.

-- Increase or decrease in sexual desires.

-- Agitation for no apparent reason.

-- Belligerency for no apparent reason.

-- Inability to carry on a conversation.

-- Repeating same statement over and over again.

-- Disoriented as to time or place.

It's difficult to understand how patients can exhibit many of the above symptoms and still be able to sit down and play bridge in an acceptable manner. Sometimes they are able to retain some skills in woodworking, sewing or other tasks for a while after the illness is noted. Then gradually these skills are lost, a little at a time.

Typically, when it comes to the memory loss of Alzheimer's disease, the most recent events are the first to go. The patient will function very well in familiar tasks that have been done over the years. Eventually, even familiar tasks become affected, and that is when family and associates start to notice something is wrong.

Put yourself in the patient's place: Joe and Mabel

Try to imagine how you would feel if you were the Alzheimer's patient. This is a very difficult thing to do. The following scenario may help you; as you read it, keep in mind that the loved one's behavior is typical of Stage One.

Let's make believe you are a man on his way home from work. You have had problems balancing the books lately, but the secretary found the errors and resolved the problem. You wonder why the books have been so difficult the past couple of months. On the way home from work you stop at the store to buy some supplies. You can't find your car when you come out of the store, even though you search for 15 minutes. You finally take a taxi home and plan to report the car stolen.

When you arrive, you have this conversation with your wife:

Mabel: "You're late, Joe. Did you work late?"

Joe: "Yes, dear." (To himself: I didn't know I was late. How come she thinks I'm late?)

Mabel: "I've been waiting for you to come home so I could run down to the store for a few things before supper."

Joe: "I'm tired. I'll take a short nap while you are gone."

Mabel: "Joe, where is the car? It's not in the garage!"

Joe: "It wasn't there when I came out of the store so I had to take a taxi home." (To himself: "Guess I should have told her about the car when I came home. I forgot.")

Mabel: "What do you mean it wasn't there when you came out of the store?" (To herself: "What's the matter with him? He's been acting very strange lately. How could he forget to tell me he didn't bring the car home and it might be stolen? I hope nothing is wrong with him. Something <u>must</u> be wrong. What can I do?")

Joe: "I took a taxi home." (To himself: "She seems upset about the car. What did I do with it anyhow? I wish I didn't forget so many things. I really feel stupid. How come I'm so mixed up all the time? She must think I'm crazy or something. I'm tired. Why can't I remember about the car? I'm going to take a nap.")

Mabel: "What store did you go to?" (To herself: Something is wrong with him but I don't know what it could be. I'll talk to the children about this tomorrow.")

Joe: "Downtown." (To himself: "I wish I could remember what store I was in. I seem to be getting more and more mixed up about this store and car business. I wish she would leave me alone and let me take a nap.")

Mabel: "Here's a package from the Business Center Shop. Is that the store you went to tonight?" (To herself: "My goodness. He might have had a stroke or something else. I'm going to have to take him to the doctor's tomorrow. I'm so upset! And I have to find out what happened to the car.")

Joe: "Yes, that's the store." (To himself: "That must be where I was if I have their package. I wish I could remember where I was. It frightens me when I forget things like this and it's embarrassing when she figures out I made another mistake. Where is the car? I hope I didn't do something wrong to it, but I don't remember that either. What can I do? I'm so tired and everything seems to be all mixed up today. I wish I could just go to sleep and everything would be all right when I wake up. I wish I could remember where I put the car. Maybe if I take a little vacation things will get better. She must think I'm pretty stupid. I _am_ pretty stupid. I was never like this before. I always had such a good memory and now I forget so many things and things get all confused on me. Hope Mabel doesn't tell the children about the car. That would be very embarrassing for me. Oh, I wish I knew what to do!")

Mabel: "Joe, lie down and take a nap. I'll go with Ann across the street." (To herself: "Something is wrong with Joe. I'll ask Ann to take me to the Business Center Shop to look for the car. First I have to pull myself together. I'll talk to the children tomorrow and take Joe to the doctor. What a dilemma. Oh, God, please help me! I don't know what to do.")

The above is only part of what goes on in the life of a patient with early Alzheimer's disease.

As a caregiver, you must try to learn empathy without sympathy. This means to try to understand what the patient is feeling in an objective manner, rather than subjective.

(By definition, to experience sympathy is to be emotionally affected by another's sorrows; when you experience empathy, you have an intellectual, unemotional understanding of the other.)

Try to stand back and look at the behavior as if it were a movie or TV show. Detach yourself personally and emotionally from the loved one and try to look inside him or her. Unfortunately, if you look at the situation subjectively, with sympathy, you will be unable to function adequately. You will find yourself so overwhelmed with feeling you will end up in despair.

The caregiver's role in Stage One

In the early stages of the disease, the diagnosis has been made by a medical doctor, the patient is upset because he is aware of making mistakes and forgetting things, and you, as caregiver, are beginning to lay the groundwork for the best care possible for your loved one.

I think the patient should be told as gently as possible by the primary caregiver or the doctor (or both) what is happening to him and what the future holds.

It is important to keep a door of hope open for the patient. Possibly, medical science will come up with an answer to the illness in the way of successful treatment. The primary caregiver must engage the patient's full confidence. Also, keep in mind he or she will remember and understand only part of what is explained at this time.

I must emphasize that the caregiver MUST come to terms with the fact that the patient is ill, and not expect the patient to function properly. One of the most serious mistakes caregivers make is to expect their loved ones to function as they always have because they still look the same.

Caregivers often allow themselves to become angry or frustrated when the patient does something off the wall. This is when the caregiver most needs an objective attitude toward what is happening, and a strong sense of humor.

Remember, you are going through a grieving process. You are beginning to realize you are losing the essence of a loved one more and more as the disease progresses.

Perhaps it's the denial part of grieving that makes caregivers so prone to anger and frustration. Don't chastise yourself when you find yourself doing this. Take a minute to review your priorities. You will find yourself relieved, happier and better able to cope with the problems at hand.

Don't forget that you are doing a wonderful thing by taking care of your loved one. This can be especially difficult when you look around and see others having a good time and here you are, in over your head with problems. Just pat yourself on the back and remember you are not alone. When you find yourself feeling like this, ask someone to mind your patient and get away for a while. Go to a movie, eat, walk -- whatever will help you.

Practical matters

I strongly recommend that an Alzheimer's patient wear an identification bracelet. If he is separated from you accidentally, he may not be able to tell the authorities who he is or where he lives. The bracelets are nominally priced, and the peace of mind they provide is well worth it.

I have also seen Alzheimer's patients with wallets full of important identification and credit cards. The Medicare card and other hospital cards are so important they should NOT be carried by the sick patient. Replace them with other ID cards that are not as valuable. The patient will be happy with almost any cards, and you will be able to protect the important ones from loss.

One of the first things the primary caregiver should do after the doctor has made the diagnosis is to visit a reputable lawyer. It is important, while the patient is still competent, to protect his best interests and those of his family. If the patient owns any assets (real estate, cash, other valuables), these must be protected.

It might be wise for the caregiver to visit the lawyer alone the first time for advice on what needs to be done. This will make it easier to explain, later, to the loved one.

Unfortunately, the initial reaction of the patient when told the need of a lawyer is often a vehement and resounding "NO!" If this happens, let the matter rest a short while and then introduce the idea again. Sometimes the loved one won't listen to a family member but will accept advice from a close friend or business associate. You may find that this is the best avenue.

Another issue that should be addressed right away is the patient's car and drivers license. The doctor should decide if the patient is competent enough to drive. Of course you don't want to remove privileges or pleasures from your loved one. But you also have to keep in mind that a car is a powerful machine, capable of injuring or killing the patient and others.

Keep in mind that a drivers license is more than just a license to drive. It signifies independence. The ramifications of having to forfeit it can be humiliating and painful. You must be as gentle as possible with your loved one when discussing this. However, it is of utmost importance, and must be dealt with before there is a mishap.

Caregivers often find a vanishing set of friends and relatives who are "busy" and unable to visit when the onset of Alzheimer's disease first becomes apparent.

You must realize that these friends and relatives run a gamut of emotional distress, much the same as the immediate family is experiencing.

Their friend or relative is not acting normally, they are deeply concerned and don't know what to say or do.

And what <u>do</u> they do? They stay away. We all are afraid of the unknown. But if the caregiver reaches them with information about the disease, opens the problem to discussion and understanding, and requests assistance early on, the results will often be more favorable than if it is all kept secret. It's not really a secret anyhow. It's just denied or not discussed.

Finally, find a good Alzheimer's caregiver's support group in your area and go to the meetings. Even if you don't feel the need of support now, you will as the illness progresses. Don't allow yourself to think you can do it alone and then find yourself overwhelmed and frazzled.

A caregiver's checklist for Stage One
The following is a list of important things for the caregiver to do while the patient is in Stage One:

-- Establish within the family who will be the primary caregiver.

-- The primary caregiver must develop a realistic perspective on the job ahead, and learn to have an objective manner.

-- Decide which family members will assist the caregiver and determine how much of the caretaking they are able to do.

-- Speak with the extended family (brothers, sisters, etc.) and ask if they will be able to assist with the patient in some way. Suggest one day a week or one weekend a month.

-- Obtain an identification bracelet for the loved one.

-- Remove important ID, hospital and credit cards from the patient's purse or wallet for safekeeping.

-- Establish good rapport with the patient's medical doctor.

-- Consult the doctor concerning the patient's ability to drive.

-- Establish legal protection for the loved one and his or her immediate family.

-- Learn all you possibly can about the illness so you can deal with it in the best possible way.

-- Try to teach relatives and friends about the illness so they will understand what is happening to the patient and be of some help to the primary caregiver.

-- Find a good support group in your area and attend the meetings.

Chapter Four
Preventing Catastrophic Reactions

I would like to discuss catastrophic reactions with you in more detail. (We touched on the subject earlier in Chapter One.)

Many caregivers never see a catastrophic reaction, but I feel you should be forewarned. You should be aware of what can happen and know ahead of time how to avoid it.

According to Webster's Dictionary, "catastrophic" is synonymous with disastrous, calamity and misfortune; it means a disturbance of the existing order of things.

A person with Alzheimer's disease has a catastrophic reaction when he or she loses all control and becomes totally irrational.

The patient screams, yells, punches, kicks and does many other terrible things he would not normally do. In this irrational state he is able to do serious injury to himself and others.

It can be difficult to restrain a patient who is having a catastrophic reaction. I have seen five people hold down one skinny little lady.

Obviously, you must try to avoid a catastrophic reaction if at all possible. Keep in mind that you are dealing with a person whose brain is damaged in certain areas, yet who also has some areas of the brain still functioning.

You have to try to reach the part of the brain that is intact. Then lead the patient, gently and slowly, down the path you want him to take.

If you go too fast you will increase the fear, frustration and anger that have built up within him, and you will get it all back in the form of a volcano.

There are no hard and fast rules to follow. Some things work like a charm for one person but don't help at all for others.

You should do whatever it takes to avert a catastrophic reaction, but never make the mistake of doing it in anger.

If you allow yourself to become angry, you have lost perspective on the situation. You have forgotten the need to put the sick one first. You won't be able to think well when you are angry, and you need to be able to plan what you say and do. Take a deep breath, start over, and do your best.

Keep the patient calm

As I mentioned before, when you see a mood escalating in a patient, try to change the train of thought or activity immediately. This is essential. If you allow the patient to become too excited, it will be that much more difficult to calm him down.

As the caregiver, you must be sensitive at all times to your loved one's mood and react accordingly. He must remain your primary concern. Everything else takes a back seat, and everything revolves around him.

Of course, this is easy to say and not so easy to do. Unfortunately, if you don't keep the patient primary you will end up with problems that easily could have been avoided.

Keep in mind that the patient never plans a catastrophic reaction. It is simply a mood that escalates and gets out of hand. Because your loved one has damaged brain cells, he is unable to fully verbalize feelings. The patient's judgment is impaired and he has forgotten many important things.

He is confused by all that is happening, knows he is losing control, and doesn't know what to do about it. Like a snowball, the reaction just grows.

If you see escalating moods in your loved one frequently, speak to his physician about it. He may want to order medications that will minimize mood swings.

Sometimes a patient will get an incorrect idea fixed in his head. Often the idea is slightly paranoid in nature ("someone is plotting against me," or "someone took something of mine.")

Within the sick mind this one mistaken idea remains, and any amount of reasoning and discussion will not shake it.

Unbelievably (and unfortunately), the patient can retain this incorrect bit of information for a long time. We cannot explain this but we see it happen frequently. And this often is the basis of the start of a catastrophic reaction.

I must emphasize that reasoning will not help. Even when you prove it isn't so, your loved one will cling to the mistaken idea and no amount of talking will convince him he is wrong. Your best hope is to get him busy or talking about something else, and hope the short term memory loss will help him forget his error, at least temporarily.

If, for example, you are in a sitting area, you might suggest having a cup of tea and a slice of cake, and then go and get it. Ask the patient to cut the cake or get the plates.

In other words, distract your loved one from the source of irritation. If this fails, you might excuse yourself to go to the bathroom. When you return, initiate a different activity.

Sometimes the short term memory loss is a help to you, and this could be one of those occasions.

I saw a woman scream and yell, then walk across a room to pick up a book. In less than a minute she returned to the person she had been screaming at to show her something in the book. The anger and the incident had been erased from the patient's mind by the disease. You can't always count on this but it does happen occasionally.

Sometimes it helps if you, yourself, adopt different moods. Start by explaining what you want from your patient. If that doesn't work, try coaxing. "Sweet talk" the patient. You might say, for example, "Yes, that's right, but could we do this first, and then we'll do that?" Always try to agree with the patient by saying "Yes, but..." This avoids disagreement and saves face for someone who ends up doing something other than he or she had intended.

If you are still up a creek, take a firm stand. You might even start to chastise to see if that will help. If it doesn't, a neutral attitude may lead to success.

We mentioned hugs earlier and they deserve to be mentioned again. They frequently work--quite unexpectedly.

An animal can be helpful. The presence of a dog or cat can change a mood immediately and sometimes will remove the entire problem. Petting a cat or dog often is as soothing to the one doing the petting as it is for the animal. Pets also inject a playful mood. What a wonderful distraction from a big problem!

Keep the patient busy

Another tactic is to channel the energy of the escalating mood, before it reaches crisis proportions, into something constructive.

You might say, "I'm going to clean the house now. Would you vacuum for me?" Most of the time you will get a favorable reaction and you will have aborted a big problem. You could just as easily suggest washing dishes, sweeping the sidewalk or many other household chores. Or, "Let's take a walk or a ride in the car."

Establish a routine and try to stay within its bounds. If the routine must be changed, tell the patient. He may not understand all of it completely, but some will be understood, and that might be enough to engage his cooperation. Be direct with the patient and tell him what is going on even if you don't think he will understand. He may grasp all or part of what you are explaining to him.

Use your imagination and plan ahead so you will be ready when a catastrophic reaction begins to build. Learn to invent games or things to do.

It helps to have one room that is a "safe room." Make it comfortable, with an easy chair, a bed, no sharp furniture edges, and no areas where the patient could fall and injure himself. Include magazines with interesting pictures and boxes containing colorful scarves, belts, soft stuffed animals, and wood pieces that can be put together like a puzzle.

Perhaps include such things as paper, colored markers, paint for painting pictures, and shells and other items that might be glued on paper for decoration.

It doesn't matter if the patient makes mistakes, if the activity keeps him or her interested and happy. Plan on some "together time" and do a craft together.

I have seen one patient keep busy folding laundry for an hour. As the patient folds items, you can unfold them put them back in the pile to be done again (don't let him see you doing this). Keep towels that need folding available for just such situations.

Another activity many people enjoy is cooking. Work with your loved one and let him measure the ingredients for a cake or cookies, peel potatoes or carrots, and/or make a salad. This keeps the patient's hands and mind busy on a task with instant reward. And if he makes a mistake there is no great harm done.

Music works wonders. As we'll see in later chapters, it seems to reach even those with almost no contact with reality. Play music and let the patient dance, or dance with him for a while. (Sounds silly, doesn't it? It works.) This also provides good exercise for the patient (and caregiver).

Sing with the patient. Singing is good for everyone. It automatically elevates people's moods and relaxes them.

Get tapes of the old songs. For some reason even patients who have lost part of their speech (aphasia) will remember and sing all the words to the old songs.

Exercise is good for Alzheimer's patients, and they often enjoy the activity. If you have a garden, let the patient dig, rake or sweep. Working in a garden is gratifying to most people. Go dig in the garden with your loved one (more exercise for both of you, and you end up with pretty flowers and plants).

If tending a garden is too strenuous, get some pots, place them at waist level, and grow something pretty. Even patio tomatoes can be grown in a pot.

Play ball for a while. Just a simple game of catch is a good activity, and, again, good exercise. Exercise also will help both of you sleep well at night. That's a reward in itself.

Quick solutions

Here are a few simple things I often do when I see a patient's mood escalating. You might try them:

Whisper or speak very low. The patient has to quiet down in order to hear you.

Try to remove yourself. Walk away or sit facing the opposite direction. Make believe you are reading or sewing, but keep a wary eye. It's hard for the patient to fight if he has no one to fight with.

Put your hands behind you or in your pockets. Sometimes hands showing or touching can seem like a threat.

Make a request and a promise at the same time. For example, "Please sit down and I'll get you a soda." Then walk away. Many times by the time you come back the problem is resolved.

Sometimes just getting the patient into another room is enough to change the mood.

Wandering

One common problem that leads to a catastrophic reactions is wandering, a symptom I haven't mentioned up to this point. (We also will discuss wandering in future chapters.)

For some unexplained reason, patients frequently become restless. They want to go out when they are inside, and come in when they are outside.

They will walk around the house and touch things for apparently purposeless reasons. (If there is something you do not want the patient to touch, remove the article so the problem is prevented before it starts.)

A patient also will leave the house, walk around the neighborhood and may become lost, especially after the disease has progressed.

Obviously, this is a large concern and problem for the caregiver. I have found that if a patient is determined to go out it is safer to go with him and walk for a while.

You might suggest a ride in the car if one is available. Remember, it is easier to inconvenience yourself with a walk or a ride than to cope with a catastrophic reaction. You might even enjoy the excursion and find it an unexpected bonus for both of you.

(Of course there's no point in trying to evaluate how much trouble you may have avoided, because there is no way of knowing how excited the patient would have become.)

Summary of tips and suggestions

Here is a summary of what a caregiver might do to help prevent a catastrophic reaction:

-- Remain sensitive to the patient's mood at all times and react accordingly.

-- Distract the patient from any source of irritation.

-- Keep surroundings pleasant and cheerful.

-- Avoid conversation that is upsetting to the patient.

-- Establish a routine and try to stay within its bounds.

-- If the routine must be changed, tell the patient.

-- Try to stop the catastrophic reaction in its early stages.

-- Change the train of thought or activity immediately.

-- Get the patient busy or talking about something else.

-- "Sweet talk" the patient; always agree with him.

-- Avoid disagreement by saying, "Yes, but..."

-- Get the patient into another room.

-- Adopt different moods yourself.

-- Whisper or speak very low.

-- Remove yourself from the conflict.

-- Put your hands behind you or in your pockets.

-- Channel the energy of the escalating mood into something constructive, such as a doing a craft or folding towels.

-- Keep the patient's hands and mind busy on a task with instant reward, such as food preparation.

-- Let the patient dig, rake or sweep in the garden.

-- Play a game of catch.

-- Maintain one room that is a "safe room."

-- If the patient is determined to go out, go with him and walk for a while.

-- Suggest a ride in the car.

-- Distract the patient with a pet.

-- Play music.

-- Get tapes of the old songs.

-- Sing with the patient.

-- Give the patient a hug.

-- If a patient is wandering within the house, allow him to do so if no harm can come from it.

-- If a patient is doing repetitive behavior and no harm can come from it, allow the activity.

-- If possible, and if it is not dangerous, go along with what the patient wants to do. Chances are he or she will tire of it soon.

-- Do whatever is necessary to prevent a catastrophic reaction, but never act in anger.

Chapter Five

Stage Two: Acceptance

S tage Two is a fuzzy area. I call it Acceptance but there are others who may disagree with me.

As I mentioned, some patients are able to develop insight when they first become ill. Some areas of the brain are affected in the beginning, but most of the brain is still functioning well. The caregiver should strive to encourage use of the highest function.

It is hard to figure out what part of the brain's reasoning and judgment are intact, and what part has been destroyed, because thoughts are abstract. It is easy to observe that your loved one can't count any more, but how do you know if he realizes what is happening?

Many times a patient will say something like, "Why don't I remember that?" or, "I know I always forget things, and I don't know why, because I always had such a good memory."

If you simply explain that he is sick, reassure him that if he forgets you will remind him, and tell him you will take care of whatever is necessary, he will accept your answer. He is aware something is wrong and is willing to hand over responsibility to someone he can trust. It is a great comfort for the patient to know he has a loved one who cares enough to share his terrible problems.

Of course, you should remember the patient is going to forget that he has placed his trust in the caregiver's hands. He will have to be reminded and reassured many times.

This takes a great deal of patience, as well as understanding of the disease, on the part of the caregiver. The tenth time you have virtually the same conversation you may find yourself exasperated.

This is when you have to remind yourself that the patient is someone you have loved dearly for many years, and who is no longer responsible for himself or anyone (or anything) else. The more you understand the disease the easier it will be, both for you and your loved one.

Stage Two symptoms

In addition to the long list of symptoms for Stage One (see Chapter Three), add these:

-- Some areas of the brain are impaired, others are not.

-- The patient begins to accept the fact that he is sick.

-- Accepts reassurance from the caregiver.

-- May become depressed and withdrawn.

-- Moves from one stage to another throughout the day.

Betty accepts her illness

I remember one lady I had as a patient when I worked in a hospital. I'll call her Betty.

When I arrived at work, the morning report stated she had had a fall between the bathroom and her bed. There were no injuries noted.

On my initial rounds, I stopped to talk with Betty and to double check that there were no injuries. I asked her if she could tell me what had happened. She said, "Yes, but I don't know if you will understand."

I told her, "Try me."

"My husband died."

"I can share that with you, because my husband died, too."

She then said, "I still talk to him as if he were still alive." I told her I could understand that, too, because you can talk to someone spiritually, even though he is deceased.

She continued, "Well, coming back from the bathroom I was talking to him and holding his arm. I forgot he was dead and I leaned on him. After I fell I remembered he was dead."

Betty could remember the fall, and she realized her mistake in thinking her husband was still alive. I believe she learned to accept her illness at that point. Betty had wonderful insight into her situation and was coping with it the best way she could.

Two patients who could laugh about it

I once had a neighbor, Bea, who lived alone. I was very fond of her. Bea's husband had died many years before and she managed rather well alone. She had early Alzheimer's disease and I would check on her frequently to see that she had no problems.

One afternoon I stopped by after work and noticed she was all dressed up, with make-up on and her hair in place. I said "Oh, you look so pretty. Where are you going?"

She looked at me with a sweet smile and said, "Well, I'll tell you. I was so warm this afternoon that I went in and took a bath. Then I got out my clothes and got all fixed up nice. After I got all dressed up I realized I had no place to go. I decided to just sit here and look pretty for the rest of the day."

She knew she forgot. She was aware of it. Fortunately, she was able to laugh at herself. Needless to say we went downtown for a soda. A sweet, pretty lady like that deserved a place to go and to have fun.

Another little lady, whom I'll call Nancy, took me by surprise one day. She was in a retirement home in a room she shared with her husband. I had entered the room with their medications. While talking with them I asked Nancy if she had any children. She gave me a quizzical look, turned to her husband and asked, "Do we have children?"

He assured her they had two children.

Then she asked me, "What does that pill do to me?" When I told her it was her vitamin pill she laughed and said, "Young lady you're about 50 years too late." She had forgotten her children, yet she knew who her husband was and she still retained her fine sense of humor. I think she was aware of her loss of memory and had accepted the fact. She was able to laugh at the situation.

Lucy learned to not worry about it

I recall another lady, whom I'll call Lucy, who just about broke my heart. We were in a day care setting and she decided she didn't want to wait for transportation home; she would walk instead. This was an impossible situation, one that I could not allow.

Her mood escalated rapidly, and I was afraid we would end up with a catastrophic reaction. Naturally I wanted to avoid this if at all possible.

In her anger she finally said, "I can walk home without getting lost. I know every inch of Omaha."

In desperation, I picked up a newspaper and was able to prove to her we were in Miami.

She blanched and started to shake. I put my arms around her and let her cry a little. Lucy not only allowed this closeness but welcomed it. She knew she had troubles, but also that she had a friend.

Yet I sensed I had broken her spirit. A few minutes later I asked her to help me with a project. She came in a very docile manner, settled down quietly and seemed to be content to help me.

Before she went home that night she said, "My brain doesn't remember things like it used to, but I'm not going to worry about it." Lucy had some insight into her problem and had accepted the situation for the time being.

For several weeks after that she appeared depressed. She withdrew from most activities and read or slept most of the time. Repeated attempts to bring her into conversation would be answered with, "I don't feel like talking now," and she would bury her head in a book.

Many times during the day I would ask Lucy a question or invite her to help me with something, and I always received a negative answer.

I realized she needed time alone, but continued to invite her; when she said no I would tell her I would save a chair for her if she changed her mind.

One day my efforts were rewarded. Lucy came to me and asked, "Which chair did you save for me?" She received a big hug and a chair -- and I have to admit tears were in my eyes.

This illustrates a large area of judgment every caretaker faces: When to insist and when to allow. I suggest you do whatever works, and practice trial and error.

I am often asked how I know if a patient is aware or unaware of something, and how I know if he or she is in the acceptance stage.

There is no hard and fast answer. You have to test the patient's mood and trust your intuition. You will not always be right, but you should not let this upset you. Look for humor in the situation and try to laugh about it. Then start all over again.

I believe Lucy exemplified a near-catastrophic reaction, Stage One behavior (aware of some errors), and Stage Two behavior (acceptance) -- all in a very short span of time.

Inside Lucy's damaged mind

Are you able to empathize with your Stage Two patient? Empathy comes from understanding what is going on in a person's mind.

For example, here is what Lucy might have been saying to herself:

"I don't know what place this is. I think I'll go home. Why won't that woman let me leave, anyhow? Who does she think she is? I don't know who she is, either. She's pretty bossy. She said I can't leave. I'm leaving, whether she says so or not. She can't keep me here. I'll just push past her and go out the door. I don't know where I am and I don't want to stay any longer. I'll go no matter what she does. Why doesn't she move and let me go? She says I'll have a ride home later. I want to go now. I don't want to yell like this. I know I'm yelling and I can't stop. She said I'm not in Omaha. Where does she think this is? Why is she saying I can't walk home? I can walk far if I have to. She keeps talking to me. I wish she would shut up and go away and leave me alone. She wants me to look at a newspaper. I just want to leave and go home. I don't know this place and want to get out of here now.

"Oh, my goodness, this is Miami. The paper said so and so did that lady. How did I get to Miami? Where am I? I wish I could stop shaking. I'm all mixed up. If I'm in Miami I can't go home alone. I don't know where I am. That lady seems to know where I am. She's hugging me even though I yelled at her. Oh, I think she's really a nice lady even though I didn't think so before. Maybe I'll stop shaking in a few minutes. I wish I wouldn't cry in front of all these people. What am I going to do? I'm all alone and don't know where I am. I'll just stay with this lady. She seems like she might be OK. She seems to know where we are and that's a help. She said she would get me a cup of coffee and I'll just sit in this chair and maybe then I can remember where I am and things won't be so mixed up.

"I'll just stay here and see if she really gets me a ride home. I seem to be having a lot of things get mixed up and confused lately. I can't remember everything like I used to. I used to be able to remember everything. I feel stupid. What good am I? I don't know what to do. I'll just do the best I can and maybe that nice lady will help me. Guess I won't remember everything any more. Maybe I'll help that lady with her work later but now I just want to sit and try to think."

When stages combine

Even though you try to understand what your loved one is able to do or think, you will never know exactly what or how much has been damaged in his thinking process.

You may realize your loved one is hallucinating and is unable to participate in any formal activity, and then he surprises you. Something totally intact comes through.

All patients can move from one stage to another and back again many times a day. Just like anyone, their moods and degrees of alertness vary widely, going up and down with meals, fatigue or stimulation. An Alzheimer's patient maintains these normal variations in mood, yet at the same time suffers the affects of brain deterioration.

Why are some patients able to function so well in some areas and not at all in others? Here is an analogy that may help:

If you drop a glass on the floor it will shatter. When you pick up the broken glass there are small and large pieces. Some are so crumbled that you have to sweep them up. When you try to put the glass together again, there are pieces missing.

The dropped glass is like a brain affected by Alzheimer's disease. Some areas are crumbled, some pieces (large and small) are intact, and some pieces are missing altogether.

Beth could not accept her illness

Beth is an example of someone who mixed stages, yet never really experienced Acceptance. She was in Partial Care (which we will discuss in detail in Chapter Seven). Her husband helped her dress, put on her makeup and fixed her hair. When she tried to tell us something, she would lose her thought mid-sentence. She would also use incorrect words at times. Beth was at times acutely aware of this, at other times unaware.

Beth would get confused following simple directions. For example, when we were cooking, we put the canister of flour, a measuring cup and a spoon in front of her, and asked her to measure one cup of flour for the cake. She was unable to do it. She tried, and knew she was doing it wrong. When we put the spoon in her hand and guided it to the flour she would then put a spoonful of flour into the cup. But she was unable to follow through with the next spoonful, and we would have to guide her hand again.

She would often say, "I can't do it." When we reassured her that there was no hurry, and that we would help her, she would respond with a smile and do it with us.

She knew she had Alzheimer's disease, yet never came to terms with the fact. She frequently cried and would say, "My husband is so good, he deserves a better wife than I can be to him."

I used to wish for her sake she would lose some of her awareness and become more accepting. I knew time would take care of this, but also that Beth was going through a very difficult part of her illness. She needed all the support she could get in order to maintain her self-esteem.

A caregiver's checklist for Stage Two

In addition to the suggestions recommended in earlier chapters, these are especially important during Stage Two:

-- Reassure and comfort the patient, repeatedly, with words and hugs.

-- Give the patient time alone if he or she needs it.

-- Test the patient's moods and practice trial and error.

-- Keep your sense of humor.

Chapter Six

Stage Three: Unaware

As the disease progresses, your loved one will be less aware of his or her difficulties, and will be less able to prevent, cope with or otherwise hide problem behavior.

Not surprisingly, this is a difficult time for both patient and caregiver. Brain damage becomes more apparent, and patients may not recognize their own homes or even their caregivers.

As a caregiver, you have to exercise judgment all day every day. You will find things that work some of the time will fail at other times. At times you will have to be firm, at other times gentle. Above all, you must always be kind.

Many times making promises will help ("if you do this then I'll do that"). But you must be sure you keep your promises and never lie to your loved one. Keep in mind that patients do remember some things, and a caregiver must strive to maintain a patient's confidence. If, for example, you are going out and leaving your loved one in someone else's care, tell him. Don't sneak away. He may not like it, but he will know (at least for the moment) that you can be trusted.

Expect the stages to mix, which will lead to behavior that might surprise you.

I recall, for example, a man whom I assumed was unaware. Tom walked around all day, moving chairs and tables about the room for no apparent reason. He couldn't sit still more than two minutes and was unable to hold a conversation. One day I asked him how he was doing, and much to my surprise he replied, "I'm eating humble pie." When I asked what he meant, he explained, "I used to know all the answers and now I don't seem to know any answers." I was amazed so much insight could come from someone who appeared to be totally unaware of his surroundings.

Stage Three symptoms:
In addition to symptoms present in earlier stages, these may also become noticeable:
-- The patient is unaware of making errors, most of the time.
-- Unaware of "filling in" with sounds instead of words.
-- Unaware of losing a train of thought.
-- Wandering, sometimes for hours, until tired.
-- Loss of reasoning powers.
-- Aware only of the present (now).
-- Unaware of what happened yesterday.
-- Unable to plan tomorrow.
-- Can't sit still.
-- Unaware of surroundings.
-- Confusion that leads to anxiety.
-- Asks the same question repeatedly.
-- Unable to retain or process information.
-- Loss of short-term memory.
-- Unable to hold a conversation.
-- Knows you are talking to him, but doesn't know who you are.
-- A few brain pathways and personality traits remain intact.

The patient's viewpoint

Try to imagine what it's like to be mixed up and not certain of your surroundings, yet you try to function properly. Let's say you're in a room with other people. You might say to yourself:

"What room is this? Am I home? Am I visiting? Have I been here before? I wish I knew where I was. It would be so much easier. It looks familiar, but I'm not positive I know where I am. What is that lady's name? She called me Mother but I don't remember any children. Maybe she just calls all ladies Mother. She keeps talking to me, but what is she saying? I'll just walk around a while and try to figure out what to do. She doesn't want me to walk around. I don't know what to do. I wish I could remember this place. If I could just find a chair I could sit down for a while. She told me to sit. Who is she anyhow? Where does she want me to sit? Why can't I get my coat off? It feels like it's stuck. What is she doing to the front of my coat? Oh, that's right. I forgot to open the buttons. I'll just smile and say thank-you to that lady. She called me Mother again. Maybe I am her mother. Wish I could remember. Thank goodness she found me a chair. I'll sit a while. I'm going to see what's over there. Oh, my, she wants me to sit again. I did sit. OK, I'll sit. I'll just be quiet so I won't make another mistake. Gee, I wish I knew where the bathroom is. Oh, I'll just wait. But it hurts. I really have to go. Maybe if I tell that lady she will help me. If I get up she'll tell me to sit down again. I better tell her."

What a terrible situation to find yourself in! An Alzheimer's patient in Stage Three experiences this all day, every day. It's almost too much to imagine.

Unaware and filling in

Stage Three patients often lose the ability to find the right words when speaking. Some will stop when they can't find the word; others will fill in with sounds that are not words. They know what they are trying to say, and it can be difficult for a caregiver to discover if they know they are filling in or if they are unaware of it.

For example, one of my patients said all the wrong sounds when playing with me. I suspected he was doing the sounds on purpose because he knew he was unable to find the right words. His sense of humor was still intact even though his vocabulary had been severely weakened.

If you find yourself in a similar situation, what should you do? Make an effort to guess what the patient is trying to tell you. Sometimes his body language and the situation will help you. If the patient tells you your response is not what he wanted, ask a double-bind question: "Would you like to eat or take a walk now?" rather than "What do you want?" The patient thinks he just told you.

If you are unable to figure out what the patient is trying to say, try changing the topic gracefully: "Why don't we have some lunch now?" Most of the time the patient will follow your suggestion. His short term memory loss is now in your favor. Frequently he will forget what he was trying to tell you.

Another graceful way of easing a patient's tension when you don't understand is to tell him something. This might sound, at first, like it would cause more frustration. It might at times, but most of the time it distracts the patient enough to change his train of thought completely, relieving the problem.

For example, you might say, "I don't know where I left my glasses. Have you seen them?" This should distract the patient enough to forget he was trying to tell you something. If that doesn't help, you might simply say, "I don't understand you now. Why don't you tell me again later?" That puts the question on hold for a while. And maybe later the patient will be able to tell you or show you what he was trying to say.

Try to save face for your loved one at all times. Keep in mind that most of the time he is unaware of his errors.

Loss of train of thought

A man called Carl greeted me after I returned from vacation with, "Where were you? I missed you."

I was surprised he remembered I had been gone. I replied, "I was on vacation and just got back."

Carl replied, "How far back?" He was totally unaware he had lost his train of thought. I ignored the wrong answer and invited him to come and have a soda. He agreed and away we went.

Yet Carl's awareness was only partially gone. He was able to notice errors other patients made, and would give me a knowing look and half smile. He then would make his best effort to assist them in what ever activity was going on at the time.

How can you tell what a patient understands, and what part of his information processing has been destroyed? You can't. The best you can do is give it a calculated guess.

Loss of logic, reason and memory

Patients in Stage Three also lose their powers of logic and reasoning. They are unable to comprehend abstract thoughts and are unaware of the loss. When a patient is not doing what you wish, you cannot use logic to persuade him. It doesn't work.

You can no longer say to the patient, "If you do something today, then tomorrow we will do something else." The patient knows what is going on right now, period. He doesn't know he is unaware of what he did yesterday or that he is unable to plan tomorrow. He might remember bits and parts, but for all practical purposes, he only knows "now."

Because short term memory has been seriously affected by the disease, the patient is constantly in unfamiliar surroundings. He doesn't know where the bathroom is or where he left his sweater.

This also explains why patients will ask the same question every few minutes. They become anxious about a situation they don't understand, ask their caregiver and the caregiver answers. They are satisfied and say "thank you." Yet they are unable to retain the information, and repeat the question.

The reason for this seems obvious, but can be difficult to understand. I've seen caregivers shake their heads in disbelief at how rapidly the information leaves the patient. Like water going through a strainer, the information is never really processed. There is no part of the brain left in that area to receive the information. So like a strainer without a bowl under it, the information just passes through and is lost.

Not surprisingly, the need to continually repeat information and to answer the same questions over and over often creates impatience or anxiety on the caregiver's part. You must exert great patience and always keep in mind that memory loss is not your loved one's fault.

Anxiety

Anxiety is very common in Alzheimer's patients who are mostly unaware, yet also to some extent aware. For example, a patient may know you are talking to him but may not know who you are. This causes great confusion within the patient, and in turn, the confusion causes anxiety.

Anxiety is frequently the cause of catastrophic reactions, which we discussed in detail in Chapter Four. You want to make a sincere effort to keep the patient's anxiety level down, not only for his or her comfort (and yours), but also to avoid a catastrophic reaction.

Be on guard at all times to avoid doing or saying anything in front of your loved one you wouldn't do or say if you knew he was fully cognizant. Something, even in the sickest brain, is still working. You don't want to cause greater injury than has already been done.

Sarah danced away her anxiety

I remember a woman, whom I'll call Sarah, who was always very anxious about her husband coming to pick her up from day care at the end of the day. Even though her husband was a reliable person who never missed, her anxiety and upset grew to fever pitch as the day progressed.

Sarah vacillated through Stages One, Two and Three throughout the day. She was often very aware of making mistakes and would say, "I know I'm wrong, but would you tell me anyhow?" And then, "I'm afraid he won't come." She would have tears in her eyes and be almost unable to think about anything else. She wanted to sit and look out the window all day, "in case he comes early."

In this sort of situation, what should a caregiver do? Reassure, reassure, reassure. Give frequent hugs. And promise to stay with her until her husband comes.

Also, try to divert attention away from any obsession or source of anxiety. We would request Sarah's assistance in some little job, or perhaps a craft. To our delight, she would sometimes really get into the craft and enjoy doing it.

Other times she would say, "I'd like to help you but I have to stay here." When this was her response, we would take a firm stand and pleasantly tell her that we understood she wanted to look out the window, but it was a rule that we all had to help with the craft or activity. She would come reluctantly, yet before long she would be happily involved in what she was doing.

Our payoff came one day when we were dancing with the group and singing and Sarah said, "Why should I sit and wait for him when I can dance like this?" When you are a caregiver, much of your satisfaction comes from having made someone better, happier or more contented.

I recall another incident with Sarah that illustrates verbal loss, word substitution and loss of reasoning ability. We were talking about waiting for her husband and she said, "I sure wish we had a geography book so we could look up where he is and call him." She substituted "geography" for "telephone" and reasoned she could find out where he was by looking in a book.

Like many patients in Stage Three, Sarah was at least partly aware (of her unnecessary anxiety about her husband), yet also was totally unaware (of the word substitutions she used).

Unaware and wandering

Many patients in Stage Three wander, yet are unaware that they are wandering. It is a waste of time to try to get a patient who is wandering to sit still or lie down. It's almost as if there is a motor inside that demands activity. Try to channel this activity in a manner that is favorable for both caregiver and patient. With a little effort you can focus this energy into something productive, such as gardening or a game of ball.

If you approach this properly, you can get ironing, vacuuming and many other household chores completed, and your patient will be tired. This gives both of you a rest. Since the patient is unaware and also has short-term memory loss, you may have to re-engage him in the favorable activity frequently. Sometimes he will need you with him to continue the activity.

If the patient is simply wandering and not doing any harm, let him wander. After a while he will get tired and stop. I have watched people wander for hours almost non-stop. You can interrupt them for a drink or snack, but they will go back to wandering if that is their theme of the day.

This is one reason why no one should take care of an Alzheimer's patient alone over the long term. The caregiver needs a respite. Without respite, unfortunately, you stand a good chance of developing a diminished feeling of well-being and even serious health problems.

I once watched a patient who was unaware he was wandering, and who was picking up furniture for no reason, smile pleasantly and hold a door open for someone. Was holding the door a conditioned reflex that didn't involve a thought process? I don't think so. I believe many ingrained personality traits stay intact, following old worn pathways to the brain, in spite of the ravages of Alzheimer's disease.

Ed is persuaded to return

A private van brought Alzheimer's patients to the day care center where I worked. One day I watched as one man (whom I'll call Ed) got off the van quietly, did an about face, and headed toward the street.

I knew Ed was totally unaware of his problems and I knew I could not expect reasoning to help. So I just followed him and asked him where he was going. He said he was going home. I knew he had no idea where he was and was just wandering.

I asked him, if I came along, would he get me a cup of coffee when we got home? He assured me he would. I was now a friend walking home with Ed. The van driver noted the two of us leaving, and after discharging the other patients, followed us.

When the driver caught up to us I said to Ed, "Look at the bus. Why don't we take it instead of walking?" He said he thought that was a good idea, got on the bus willingly and we returned to the day care center.

When we got there I asked Ed, "Why don't we go in and get a cup of coffee?" Again, he agreed with my suggestion. We went in, had (decaf) coffee, and spent a peaceful day together. Wasn't I lucky to have his short term memory loss on my side?

Sometimes you have to walk a fine line when it comes to deciding to do what is right. Ed was in Stage Three, he was unaware, and he had no powers of reasoning. In this case I believe a catastrophic reaction was avoided.

A caregiver's checklist for Stage Three

In addition to suggestions included in earlier chapters, you may find these particularly helpful during Stage Three:

-- Make an effort to guess what the patient is telling you.

-- Read the patient's body language.

-- Ask questions that offer choices (not, "What do you want?")

-- Use the patient's short term memory loss to your advantage.

-- Help the patient save face.

-- Ignore wrong answers.

-- Put the patient's question on hold if you don't understand it.

-- If you don't understand what the patient is telling you, diffuse the tension by telling him something.

-- Keep the anxiety level down to prevent a catastrophic reaction.

-- Channel wandering into a more productive activity.

-- Stay with the patient during an activity.

-- Expect to have to re-engage the patient in the activity frequently.

-- Don't try to get a restless patient to sit still or lie down.

-- Seek respite for your own health and well-being.

-- Do not use logic or try to reason with the patient.

-- Don't do or say anything in front of a patient that you wouldn't do if he was fully cognizant.

Chapter Seven
Stage Four: Partial Care

When your loved one was in the early stages of the disease, he showed memory lapses which became more frequent and noticeable. He displayed errors in judgment, and was embarrassed and frightened.

Your loved one attempted to cover up his mistakes and was, for the most part, aware of what was happening to him. Like many patients, he may have accepted the fact that he was ill, and allowed people to assist him with daily living.

He then progressed to the point where he was aware of only some errors. All the while he gradually lost motor skills, to the point that he needed help doing tasks such as buckling his belt or tying his shoelaces.

As his decision making, recent memory and motor skills diminished, so did his ability to be self-sufficient. He appeared to be clumsy; he would trip, drop items and bump into things.

He might say, "I would like a glass of water," not because he wanted you to wait on him, but because he couldn't remember where the kitchen is. You may have discovered that if you just pointed to the kitchen he would go and get the water for himself. In other words, you could find pathways in the brain that were still usable. But even this diminished with time.

When your loved one reaches Stage Four, he will experience difficulty dressing, bathing and even feeding himself. He may forget to go to the bathroom before it is too late. You may observe bizarre behavior for which he is not responsible, and over which he has no control.

An Alzheimer's patient is really in a state of partial care from day one of the disease. He needs protection from errors in decision making and from loss of memory, even during the early onset of the disease. For our purposes, we will consider "Partial Care" to be the point at which the caregiver becomes involved in the physical aspects of caring for the patient.

Stage Four symptoms

In addition to those behaviors and symptoms found in earlier stages, a patient in Partial Care may exhibit the following:

-- Is unable to verbalize thoughts or hold a conversation.

-- Understands much of what is said but there is a loss of comprehension.

-- Is unable to follow a simple request.

-- Memory loss is more noticeable. The patient will ask questions similar to "Did we have lunch yet?"

-- Judgment is poor; poor decision making increases.

-- Disoriented as to time; merges past with present.

-- Disoriented as to place.

-- Spatial orientation is poor.

-- Coordination is poor; has a wide gait, tendency to trip.

-- Dexterity is poor.

-- Anxiety level is elevated; is nervous; cries easily.

-- May be unaware, aware and/or accepting of his own errors.

-- Has difficulty in dressing, wears wrong clothes, wears layers of clothing.

-- Has difficulty in bathing and grooming; needs assistance.

-- Exhibits restlessness, wandering and purposeless walking.

-- Uses table utensils improperly.

-- Has slight difficulty chewing and swallowing.

-- Saves useless items.

-- Has auditory and visual hallucinations.

-- Easily agitated, has wide mood swings.

-- Exhibits repetitive behavior.

-- Has bathroom accidents occasionally.

Changes in spatial orientation, coordination

It will be helpful for you to understand how your loved one's spatial orientation and coordination are changing.

Spatial orientation, in particular, is difficult to comprehend, simply because you cannot see it. It has to do with a person's relationship to the space that surrounds him, and the items in it.

When you go bowling, for example, you know the pins are at the end of the alley in front of you. If you lose your spatial orientation, you know the pins are in front of you, but you don't know which way is front. Patients will throw the ball to the side, or turn and throw it behind them.

Think about what this must be like, and try to grasp the ramifications of being without adequate spatial orientation. Imagine wanting to sit on a chair, and when you try to, you land on the floor. What happened? Your lack of spatial orientation fooled you. This can be traumatic, and it can create fear and anxiety.

The loss of spatial awareness also creates a great deal of confusion for the patient. An Alzheimer's patient will see an object in a room, yet not know how far away it is or how he can get to it from where he is standing. Many times I have suspected that the wandering we see in patients may be their way of trying to orient themselves to their surroundings.

When your loved one is hesitant about doing something, it may be due to his lack of spatial orientation. If, for example, you point to a chair across the room and ask him to sit in it, he may have difficulty in finding the chair. You may find it easier to lead him to the chair, ask him to sit, and even assist him in sitting. He may see and feel the chair, yet not be certain that the chair is really there.

If you hand a glass of water to a patient with poor spatial orientation, he may put his hand ten to 12 inches away from the glass. Or he will compensate for his difficulty by putting both hands out, spaced widely apart, and then close in on the glass. Obviously, when you hand something to a patient in this stage of the illness, you have to be sure he has it before you let go.

I have seen a patient try to climb a handrail next to a door when what he wanted was to go through the door. Perhaps his lack of spatial orientation prevented him from realizing that by walking around the handrail he could get to the door more easily. I also have seen patients try to climb over the backs of chairs in an attempt to sit in them.

Poor spatial orientation will give a patient a hesitant gait. He will tentatively feel the ground in front of him before putting his weight on the forward foot. He isn't certain the ground is there.

This also may be the reason why many patients revert to eating with their fingers instead of table utensils. They aren't sure the fork or spoon will get to their mouths, and feel more confident with hand-to-mouth activity.

Coordination is another important area of change. The motor control of our bodies is governed by our brains. When this area of the brain is affected by Alzheimer's disease, coordination is impaired. At first the impairment is hardly noticeable, but then it escalates to the point where the patient needs assistance to maintain his balance.

Combine poor memory, poor spatial orientation and poor coordination, and what do you get? A frightened, embarrassed person who is partially aware of making errors in speech and decision making, and who also has trouble walking and sitting. Furthermore, this is a very anxious person who only knows NOW. He doesn't remember what happened five minutes ago and is unable to plan five minutes from now.

You must use sensitivity to assess your loved one's needs. You want to keep your patient functioning to his greatest capability, for as long as possible. You will have to decide when to step in with assistance, and when to leave him alone to struggle. This is a large, indefinable area and you probably will make errors in judgment at times. That's OK, we all do. Just make the patient's safety your highest priority and you will do just fine.

The caregiver's dilemma

Frequently you'll find it is easier, neater and quicker to do something for a patient rather than waiting for the patient to do it himself. The caregiver walks a fine line in this area. You want him to maintain the skills he has for as long as possible, so it is often better to let him struggle a little and be successful rather than to do it for him. As the caregiver, the decision is yours. There are no hard and fast rules, so you have to do what you think is right at the moment.

Your loved one is no doubt having serious verbal problems. He is unable to find the correct word, is losing his thought in the middle of a sentence, and may be aware of his errors. How do you save face for him and lower his frustration level? Ask questions that include answers.

Instead of asking, "What color blouse do you want to wear today?" ask, "Would you like to wear the red blouse or the pink one?" In doing this, you have saved face for him, and allowed him to make a choice. Later in the illness you will have to make the decision for him, but while he is able, it is better to allow him the option.

Whatever happens, don't allow yourself to become upset. As we discussed earlier, this is the difficult part of being a caregiver: You must try hard to remain objective. Always keep in mind that your primary goal is to keep the patient safe and happy.

Don't be too hard on yourself, caregiver. You are doing a difficult job the best way you know how, and you can't do better than that. Remember to give yourself a few pats on the back as the day goes on, because you surely deserve them.

Peggy accepted her lack of spatial orientation

I recall a lady whom I will call Peggy. I believe she combined Aware, Unaware, Acceptance and Partial Care all in one lovable package.

Peggy was trying to help me water a row of potted plants. She knew what she wanted to do, and she was well coordinated. But her brain couldn't tell her to pour the water in the pot. She would pick the pot up. She would pour the water on the ground. She would try to pick the plant. And she also knew she was doing all the wrong things.

Peggy looked at me with a smile and shrugged her shoulders. She said, "That's the story of my life. I'm in the wrong pew again." For the moment, she had accepted the fact she was unable to do what she wanted to do and was laughing at herself.

I simply said, "I'll help you." I placed her hand on the watering can and directed the water flow. We both were happy to be together, and happy to be doing the job well.

Incidentally, Peggy had no recollection of watering the flowers, and repeated the very same actions the next day. For Peggy, doing almost anything was to do it for the first time.

Confusing past with present

By the time the disease has progressed this far, patients will often talk about the past as though it were the present.

People in their 90s will ask, "Have my parents called today?" In this situation, you might reorient them by saying, "Your grand-daughter will be here to pick you up at three o'clock."

A patient might tell you, "I didn't see the children come home from school." You realize he is looking for his children, who now are adults.

Often a reminder is all the patient needs to become reoriented. But it will only last a while, and then he will forget and ask about his parents, or children, again. If you find yourself fighting a losing battle, it might be better to satisfy the patient by saying, "I'll let you know when they call." Or, "I'll let you know when they get home." It depends on the situation and your own good judgment.

At the day care center, we had a patient who had been a school teacher. She would thank us profusely at the end of the day for inviting her to our house, and tell us how she had the day off from school so she could visit.

A man, whom I'll call Ben, once had worked with machinery. He would come and tell us he was going to give the machines a last check before leaving. We always thanked Ben for his trouble and allowed him to walk around the area. I think he really saw the machinery he had worked on for so many years.

Partial Care and clothing

Dressing becomes more and more difficult for patients as the disease progresses. They can't remember where their clothes are or what clothes they need.

In the early stages of the disease, if you lay clothes out on the bed, your loved one will manage to dress himself, though he may take longer than usual and not be as neat.

As the disease progresses, the patient will be less and less able to dress himself, and eventually you will dress him completely. It also will become more and more difficult for him to pull his clothes back into place when he goes to the bathroom. This may sound like a simple task, but remember, his motor skills are diminished.

Many caregivers often don't realize how difficult dressing has become for an Alzheimer's patient until he has been struggling a long while without assistance, and then presents himself in a totally unacceptable manner.

I remember one lady who usually went to the bathroom alone with no difficulty. One day she returned wearing her underpants over her slacks. Obviously, she had reached the point where she needed help, and we always went with her after that.

The caregiver needs to keep a watchful eye and step in gracefully when the need is there. And don't hesitate because your loved one is of the opposite sex. Your easiest and best bet is to simply step over your reluctance and help.

If the patient resists being helped, I find that if you just take command quietly, tell him he isn't doing it right, and you just want to fix it, he will allow you to do it.

However, you don't want to trigger a catastrophic reaction over clothing, so if worst comes to worst let the patient be poorly dressed today, then try again tomorrow. At least you tried. You can't do more than that.

As the disease progresses, it's wise to replace worn-out items in the patient's wardrobe with clothes that are easy to put on and take off: slip-on shirts, blouses and sweaters that don't need buttons; slacks and shorts with elastic tops instead of zippers and belts; shoes with Velcro fasteners instead of shoelaces. Buy things that are washable because there will be many accidental spills.

There are many men taking care of women. One man told me he felt foolish in the women's department of a store, picking out personal items of clothing for his mother. He resolved this by using mail-order catalogs.

Another unusual behavior you may notice is over-dressing. A patient, for example, might put on four pair of underpants, three dresses and several sweaters. When you ask why she is wearing so many clothes you will get a variety of answers, but I think the true answer is her confusion. She just doesn't know what to do. Or perhaps she is wearing the clothes so no one will take them.

Be sure shoes are a good fit, to avoid blisters and other painful problems. A patient's feet may swell and shoes that once fit are no longer adequate. Remember, the patient may not be able to tell you he is having difficulty.

Partial Care and hygiene

Difficulty with bathing starts with slight confusion and progresses to an inability to bathe without assistance. There are many ways to deal with this situation, but I think the easiest is to get into the shower with the patient. Sounds odd, doesn't it? But if you look at this objectively, it's not nearly as bad as it sounds. And it works.

If you feel bashful, put on a bathing suit or a smock of some sort. I learned to do it this way when I was in nursing school, working in a locked ward of a mental hospital. We wore smocks while bathing patients, and it made the whole process much easier. If the patient is able to cooperate with you, try using a shower chair and a flexible shower head.

Speaking of showers, be sure to check the temperature setting on your home's hot water heater. Set it low enough so the water will never get hot enough to burn the patient, should he turn it on when no one is watching. Scalding water can cause serious injury.

When your loved one has difficulty with an activity, many times a start will trigger a conditioned reflex or a brain pathway that is intact enough to complete the task. In other words, if you get him started in an activity, he may be able to take it from there and complete it alone.

Let's say, for example, you've asked him to brush his teeth after a meal. You know he wants to comply with your wishes, yet instead of doing it he wanders about the room. What is happening in his brain? He may be trying to remember where the bathroom is. He might even be trying to remember what his teeth are. Yes, patients can get that confused. If you take him into the bathroom, and take out the brush and toothpaste, his chances of doing it himself are very good.

Grooming is important. I believe both caregiver and patient feel better if the patient is well groomed. If you are caring for a loved one of the opposite sex, you will have to learn the grooming skills of that sex. Women will find that an electric shaver is easier to use to shave a male patient, rather than a blade. A man caring for a woman will need to learn how to groom a woman's hair and put on her makeup. Try to keep it simple. You might go to a beauty salon and ask for a short lesson on how to manage hair and makeup with minimum effort.

Partial Care and sleep

At this point of the illness, wandering is of particular concern. The patient tends to wander frequently, and will do so during the night.

One way for the caregiver to get a good night's sleep is to create a safe sleeping area. Remove all sharp tables and breakable lamps from the bedroom. Put carpeting or a non-slip rug on the floor to keep it warm and to prevent serious injury from falls. If the caregiver is sleeping in the same room, install an inside lock on the door, and put the key on an expandable bracelet that the caregiver can wear comfortably around wrist or ankle.

This way, in case of fire or other emergency, the caregiver does not have to look for a key. If you find yourself hesitant about a lock on the door, put an alarm on the door. There also are locks that can be opened from the other side of the door, if only the patient is to be confined. This enables anyone in the house to access the room in case of emergency.

Once the room is safe and secure, the caregiver can sleep without worrying about the patient wandering. You may find the patient sleeping on the floor with pillows and blankets. That's OK. The goal is for both caregiver and patient to have slept well.

Partial Care and feeding

Alzheimer's patients lose many of the niceties of polite society with the illness. They often forget how to use utensils properly and revert to using fingers. Offer a knife and fork but allow the fingers if that is what your loved one prefers.

If the patient uses his fingers, caregivers should prepare the food accordingly. For example, instead of mashed potatoes, provide boiled potatoes cut into small pieces. You can cut many other foods (fruit, cheese, meat) into finger-size pieces.

Chewing and swallowing becomes more difficult as the disease progresses, and you may want to offer only soft foods. Each patient must be assessed individually to determine his or her capabilities. It is better to stay on the safe side rather than take a chance on letting the patient choke.

Watch to make sure the patient does not overfill his mouth, and be sure tea or coffee is not too hot, in case of spills.

I remember one lady who was served sausage and eggs. We cut one sausage in pieces and left the other one whole. I don't think two minutes went by before she was turning blue and choking. She had stuffed both sausages in her mouth and of course was unable to swallow them. They were lodged in her throat, and we did manage to remove them. She recovered just fine, but what a close call we had! From then on, someone stayed with her during the entire time she was eating. Both her judgment and swallowing abilities were impaired. I recommend all caregivers learn the Heimlich maneuver, and also CPR.

I remember another partial care patient who was given a sandwich and pudding for lunch. The pudding had a spoon in it and the sandwich rested on a plate. The patient proceeded to try to eat the sandwich with the spoon, and of course was unsuccessful. When the spoon was removed and the sandwich placed into the patient's hand, the caregiver was rewarded by a beautiful smile, and the patient proceeded to enjoy his lunch.

Imagine the frustration and anger this patient would have experienced if he had been alone, hungry and unable to eat his food. Let's take a minute to look at the caregiver's role. There might be a tendency for someone to look at this patient and say, "No! That's the wrong way to eat a sandwich!" Would the patient understand this? Probably not, and it might confuse him even more. The easiest approach for the caregiver in a situation like this is to say something like, "Try it this way, it might be easier," in a soft voice. This patient also was unable to verbalize, which compounded the problem.

Incidentally, this very same patient, in less than an hour, was able to remove a chain lock fastened on the bottom of a gate with a slip hook. The only explanation I can offer is that the pathway in the brain for opening chain locks was intact, yet the hand-to-mouth coordination needed for eating had been destroyed, or partially destroyed, by the disease.

Sometimes it helps to realize the good that comes from even the simplest things you do. Let's look at what the caregiver has accomplished by handling an every day situation, such as feeding, properly. He has succeeded in giving the patient good nourishment in a peaceful, pleasant manner. He has warded off frustration and anger in the patient, and avoided a possible catastrophic reaction. He also has made his own job easier and prevented his own frustration from elevating.

Partial Care and exercise

Exercise should be a part of the daily routine for patient as well as caregiver, and ideally should benefit both. A gentle movement of all parts of the body can be accomplished with a minimum of effort. Start with the head and work down to the feet, one group of muscles after the other. This can be done sitting or standing, or half-sitting and half-standing.

Exercise should not be vigorous but done slowly and with easy motions. You might let music set the pace. When the exercise is over, both patient and caregiver should feel better for having done it.

Partial Care and outings

Outings with a partial care patient can be fun. There are many things to do.

A trip to McDonald's or some other fast food restaurant might be a pleasant change of pace. The patient will enjoy watching all the children. Other good places to go include parks, the zoo and local children's playgrounds.

Concerts and short musical performances, or parades, are wonderful and will be enjoyed by both patient and caregiver.

The ideal activity is informal and doesn't require concentration, and does not last too long. Movies are a little tedious for Stage Four patients. They are unable to follow the plot and become bored and restless.

If you notice your loved one becoming agitated or overstimulated, you will have to limit the time or places you take him. You will notice that as the patient becomes sicker these outings become less successful. Eventually most patients do better with little or no change in their environment. Expect the routine you establish for your loved one to become more limited as the illness progresses.

Partial Care and pets

Pets are soothing for the patient, and they help the caregiver, too. A pet is a friend under any circumstances, and is company at your fingertips.

Take care in choosing a pet to make sure it will fit into the daily routine of the household. Keep in mind, before you allow a pet of any kind into your home, it too will require care. I always feel that a pet brings so much happiness, it's worth the extra time and money.

Cats or a small dog are ideal for indoors, and small dogs can be trained to kitty litter. Patients will often feel satisfied just holding a small pet in their arms, or having a large one sit at their feet in the backyard. Playing with a pet, for anyone, is a pleasant diversion from every day living.

As we discussed earlier, patients mix stages. Sometimes they seem to have forgotten almost everything and relate very little to what is going on around them; sometimes they amaze you with unexpected insight. I would like to share a story about a patient and a dog that illustrates this.

Patients often become very protective of animals. We had a dog in the nursing home where I worked at one time. The dog was in during the day and had a bed outside at night. I was about to put the dog out one evening and a lady (whom I'll call Edna) asked me what I was doing to the dog. I explained I was putting the dog out in his own house. Edna wanted to see the dog's house.

She came along with me outside while I put the dog in his dog house. She thought it was too cold outside and wanted to bring the dog back in the building. I explained the dog had a dog's blanket and would be warm enough. Edna asked if the dog knew how to pull the blanket up over him.

I made the mistake of saying yes. She accepted my wrong answer, but not until she told me, "First dog I ever heard of that could pull a blanket up over himself." I was guilty of talking down to her. Edna could not remember if she had children or where she had worked, but she certainly had an open pathway to the abilities of dogs!

If you are unable to have a live pet, a stuffed animal will fill the vacancy. Stuffed animals are soft, cuddly and cute. I don't think I have ever showed a patient a stuffed animal and not received a big smile for a reward. Sometimes patients who like to hold a soft thing in their arms will relax and fall into a peaceful sleep. You might make a cute animal as one of your crafts and get double the satisfaction from it.

Partial Care and crafts

Crafts are lots of fun and can be very creative. There are many books on the topic, so I will not discuss crafts projects at length. Try to work crafts into the life of your partial care patient frequently. No matter how limited your loved one's skills, there is always something he can do with some assistance.

A patient, however, will not do a craft alone. He needs direction and someone to stay with him. Patients have difficulty following directions, so caregivers should do the craft, one step at a time, with them. The easier the craft, the better for the patient.

This reminds me of another patient (whom I'll call Fran), who also surprised me when I least expected it. The activity director in our facility had planned a craft, and had traced patterns on colored paper to be used for it. She asked me to have the patients cut out the patterns for the craft, as it was to be done the next day.

I had no idea what she planned to make. I gathered some of the patients around a table with me and showed them what needed to be cut. Fran asked me what I was going to make with the pieces we cut out. I had to admit to her that I didn't know what they would be when they were finished. Fran got up from the table and told me, "I'm not going to help you if you don't know what you are doing!"

She was right. I should have brought a sample of the finished product with me to show what we were working on. Fran did not know where she lived or where she had worked, and she couldn't remember if she had children. Yet she certainly had an open pathway to my error!

I apologized and showed her a sample of what we planned to make. Once she knew what she was doing she was more than willing to help. The next day she did not remember cutting out the patterns.

Incidentally, it's important to make sure anything you leave lying about is harmless. Patients often try to eat things that are not food, including crayons, beads, buttons and glue. This is one more reason why the caregiver should stay with the patient to protect him from danger.

Dealing with restlessness

At times I have felt like I was rounding up a bunch of pretty, colorful, busy butterflies at the beginning of an activity around a table. I would get several people seated, leave to get some others, and when I returned, the first ones had stood up again. I would just laugh and start over.

There's no point in getting frustrated about this behavior. It shows how important it is to keep your sense of humor. You might as well laugh. After all, there's not much else you can do about it.

As we discussed in earlier chapters, it helps to channel restlessness into a productive activity. Crafts, outings, exercise and pets all can be used for this, as well as chores around the house or garden.

Ben, the man I mentioned earlier who had once worked with machinery, was a patient who would get very agitated. At times he would make a great deal of noise. Ben really was lovable, but he was capable of disturbing our entire unit of patients.

If I saw him restless and walking up and down the halls I would ask him if he would help me. He always said yes. My answer to his agitation was a polishing rag for our brass hand rails and brass plates on the doors down the hall. They really were clean, but he would set about enthusiastically polishing, up and down the hall, thus dispelling his extra energy.

Ben did one side of the hall one day and after being thanked he sat down to rest. I noticed him getting restless again in about a half hour and asked him if he would do the other half for me. His answer was, "No. You didn't pay me for the other half yet." He accepted ice cream and cookies in lieu of money for his efforts.

Dealing with hoarding

An unusual behavior we see in this stage of the illness is saving things. Patients will hoard things that belong to them as well as items that are not theirs. Perhaps they have forgotten not to take things that belong to other people.

Often, these are worthless items. Patients will fill their pockets with Kleenex, paper towels, pens, silver-ware and whatever else will fit. They are not stealing, they are saving. They really think the items are theirs, and that they are valuable.

Hoarding may sound too trivial to be concerned about, but it can be a nuisance. For example, you might come home from visiting friends and find a figurine in your loved one's pocket. What are you going to do? You'll have to return it to the owner, which will likely be embarrassing,

If you anticipate this behavior, you can discretely check your loved one before leaving the friend's home and resolve the situation right then and there. In fact, at the day care, we would check some of our patients in a routine manner. No one had any ill feelings about it.

When we did crafts, scissors and crayons often disappeared. We checked a few pockets and got everything back. Checking can be done in a gentle, even humorous manner. I would ask, "Have you got anything good in your pockets?" They would look to see what they could find, and it was surprising what would come out. I then would say, "Can I put that away for you until you go home?" Usually the response was, "Oh, thank you. That would be fine." The patient would soon forget about it and there was no harm done.

Dealing with hallucinations

Many patients start to hallucinate during this stage of the illness. They will pick at things that are not there and have conversations with imaginary people. If this behavior does not agitate them, I think it is better to allow it rather than attempt to prevent the hallucinations.

In the beginning it is fairly easy to interrupt hallucinations, but as the illness progresses, it becomes more and more difficult. Sometimes a short question or statement is enough to reorient a person who is hallucinating. If it is a visual hallucination you can sometimes interrupt it by going face to face with the patient and saying something quietly.

As patients become sicker, you may have to try to interrupt a hallucination for meals or bathrooming or some other essential thing. Often a patient can be hallucinating and if you approach him with a request such as, "Will you help me water the flowers?" he will stop hallucinating and go with you. You'll find it more and more difficult to contact areas of the brain that still function properly as the patient's condition deteriorates.

Mirrors, television sets, windows and other shiny surfaces often disturb patients in this stage of the illness. They see their own reflections and think it's another person. When they mix their hallucinations with seeing a reflection, it can trigger a catastrophic reaction. You can avoid distressing the patient by removing or covering mirrors and other reflecting objects.

I once observed a woman trying to feed a picture on a dresser. We had to remove the picture. This same woman was still able to feed and dress herself and get around in a wheelchair with little difficulty. One area of her brain was injured by the disease while other areas were very much intact.

It can be distressing to watch your loved one have hallucinations. You will wonder what is going on inside his mind, and you will likely feel concerned. Here is how someone whose father has Alzheimer's might express the love, frustration and sadness many caregivers experience during this difficult time:

"What are those things you see and hear that I am unable to see and hear, my dear Dad? Sometimes I see a pained look on your face. Are you remembering a winter day when you left your warm home in order to work to support Mother and us kids? Sometimes you smile for no apparent reason. Are you remembering the look on the face of your first born child? How wonderful it would be if we could share these thoughts, both good and bad!

"And those times you are talking to someone we cannot see. Are you re-living times gone by as if they were happening again? You ask about your parents. They both have been in heaven a long time and yet you bring them back and mix them with today's world. Other times things you see make you unhappy and upset. Are you remembering the time you fell off your bike and hurt your leg, when you were small?

"Oh, how I wish I could know what was making you laugh! It might be the first time you took Mother to a dance. Isn't that a good thing to think about? What is it that you are trying to touch that I can't see? Are you back at work, or patting a little child on the head? How I wish I could read your thoughts! Sometimes you sit with your eyes closed and I know you are not sleeping. Are you seeing and hearing quiet things? How sad it is that I will never know."

Dealing with repetitive movements

Rocking or repetitive movements often present themselves during this stage of the illness. This sort of behavior can be distracting to observers. If the behavior does not agitate the patient and it is harmless to others, I would allow it.

If it disturbs others, try to place the patient in another room and check on him frequently. Sometimes in quiet surroundings the rocking or disturbing behavior will stop.

Rather than trying to stop repetitive behavior, try to engage the patient in an activity (without mentioning the unwanted behavior). Once again, practice trial and error. Sometimes one thing will work and the next time you get a poor response. Try it again, though. It might work the next time.

The caregiver's reward

Occasionally a caregiver will get an unexpected, much needed pat on the back.

I recall a lady who was in partial care. She hallucinated constantly and we had to feed her. She wandered aimlessly and we had to bathroom her. One morning, on her way into our center, she said, "This is my favorite place to be!"

We were surprised and overjoyed to hear that small sentence. There was something left in her brain we had been reaching without knowing it. All our work had not been in vain.

I frequently say to myself that if I am ever caught in a poor situation, such as that of my patients, I hope someone will treat me as well as I have treated the people I have cared for over the years. Most caregivers must have that private thought now and then.

I believe you get back from life what you put into it. Someone once said to me, "Cast your bread upon the waters and it will come back as a sandwich." What better place can you cast your good work than in the care of a loved one?

A caregiver's checklist for Stage Four:

-- Be prepared to help the patient compensate for poor spatial orientation and lack of coordination.

-- Keep a watchful eye and step in gracefully when the patient needs assistance with feeding, dressing and other activities of daily living.

-- Ask questions that include answers.

-- Replace worn-out items in the patient's wardrobe with clothes that are easy to put on and take off.

-- Make sure shoes are a good fit.

-- Check the temperature setting on your home's hot water heater to prevent scalding.

-- Create a safe sleeping area.

-- Allow your loved one to eat with his fingers and cut food into pieces he can eat easily.

-- Watch to make sure he does not overfill his mouth.

-- Be sure tea or coffee is not too hot.

-- Learn the Heimlich maneuver, and also CPR.

-- Include exercise in the patient's daily routine.

-- Choose outings that don't require concentration, and that don't last too long.

-- If you are unable to have a live pet, fill the vacancy with a stuffed animal.

-- Do crafts one step at a time with the patient. The easier the craft, the better.

-- Make sure anything you leave lying about is harmless.

-- Check the patient, routinely, for hoarded objects.

-- Allow hallucinations. When necessary, interrupt an auditory hallucination with a question. Interrupt a visual hallucination by going face to face with the patient and saying something quietly.

-- Remove or cover mirrors and other reflecting objects.

-- Allow rocking and repetitive behavior. If it distresses others, distract the patient with an activity or remove him to another room.

-- Recognize the good that comes from even the simplest things you do.

Chapter Eight
Stage Five: Full Care

There are no good stages of Alzheimer's disease for either patient or caregiver, but undeniably Full Care is the most difficult for the caregiver. Full Care probably has been attempted by one person alone more times than we can count. Unfortunately, to do so takes a tremendous toll on the caregiver. I strongly recommend that you do not attempt Full Care without assistance.

As you will see by the list of Stage Five symptoms below, the caregiver has to do all the necessities of daily living for his or her loved one. To say the least, you are coping with a difficult task. I take my hat off to you. It takes courage, determination, a lot of work and a lot of love to do the job.

I would also like to emphasize that you should not feel bad if you decide to place your loved one in a nursing care facility. This does not mean you failed. It just means you've faced the fact that Full Care is a bigger job than one person can handle.

This chapter will show you a few ways you can give the patient opportunities for pleasure and entertainment. And although it is impossible to cover nursing care completely in these pages, I will touch on a few of the basics every caregiver should know.

When your loved one reaches Full Care, you will have very little idea what is going on inside his mind. His thought processes are so fragmented and fleeting that they are beyond comprehension. You will likely find this disappointing and frustrating.

Here is an example of how a caregiver might experience the compassion, tenderness, sadness and loss typical of Stage Five:

"Mother dear, you are so quiet today. You sit in your wheel chair and just stare into space. It seems impossible that the same lady who moved about so quickly, who cooked and cleaned the house and tended us children, and who once had so much energy, could sit so still.

"Does any little part of you remember me? Can you remember any of the fun and jokes and laughter we all had together when we kids were growing up? Do you remember when your first grandchild was born? Do you remember how big Dad was, yet how gentle? You wouldn't think a hand so big and rough could have such a soft touch.

"I know you have all those memories somewhere inside of you. It's as if they are locked, and someone threw away the key. If only we could get them back out again! I pray you have only good thoughts. How I wish you could share them with us."

Stage Five symptoms:
The patient will exhibit many of the symptoms of previous stages, and also:
    -- Is unaware of surroundings.
    -- Does not recognize others.
    -- Is unaware of dangers and cannot be left alone.
    -- Has problems with eating and has to be fed.
    -- Is incontinent of urine and involuntary of stool.
    -- Is unable to do crafts or exercises
    -- Conversation is nil.

-- Does not comprehend most of what you say.
-- Has visual and auditory hallucinations.
-- Eyes have a vacant look.
-- Face has a flat look.
-- Sits or lies down most of the time.
-- Often rocks or does other repetitive motions.
-- Coordination is poor and trips or falls easily.
-- May refuse or is unable to walk or stand.
-- Is not oriented to surroundings.
-- May drool because the swallow reflex has diminished.
-- Is unable to bathe or dress without assistance.

Entertainment and activities

Patients in this stage of the illness have great difficulty following directions, and most of their pleasures are passive.

Yet they are capable of enjoying the moment. They know they are happy or sad right now. They don't remember two minutes ago nor do they anticipate the future.

Try to exercise with your loved one. If his balance is poor, have him exercise while seated on a straight backed chair. This needn't be strenuous, just move each part of the body gently. Try to do this daily for about 20 minutes. The exercise is good for circulation, body tone, appetite and a general feeling of well being.

If you have young children let them play with the patient as often as possible. Almost all older people respond favorably to young children and vice versa. The stimulation, touch and camaraderie are good for all concerned.

Animals also are good for the very ill. They are soft and cuddly and usually are received with good humor.

I think the pleasure between animals and people is mostly reciprocal. Animals tap into a natural love built into all of us. Socialization is important to the patient, and animals also help in this area.

If your loved one is not bed bound, try to get him outdoors for short periods of time, several times a day. The variation of walking and being in a different environment will be stimulating.

Wheel chair patients also reap tremendous benefits from being outdoors. I believe it also helps them sleep better at night. They seem to take a favorable turn when they smell the trees, grass and flowers. Watching the birds and squirrels is wonderful entertainment for them.

You will have to determine how much clothing your loved one needs to wear. He has lost his good judgment and will not be able to tell you if he is too warm or if he feels chilly.

Music can be magic

There is a little corner of the brain that never ceases to appreciate music. Most patients will respond in some way to music, and it is wonderful for them. I have watched patients who had no response to external stimuli move a foot in time to rhythm, or rock their heads in time with a song.

In a care facility where I once worked there was a band that frequently entertained Alzheimer's patients. When the band was finished playing for the group, some of the musicians would walk bed to bed in the wing that had the sickest patients.

It was in this wing I observed a little lady who sat day after day in a chair. Her head rested on a pillow on a table. We had tried to engage her in various activities, and her response was always poor or nil. She refused conversation and would answer questions with, "I don't know."

One day the accordionist played a song at her bedside, and there seemed to be no response. He was about to leave when her head popped up. To our amazement and delight, she requested an old song. She then put her head back on the pillow. Music had successfully reached her, and had given her something she could enjoy.

There was another lady at the same facility who was even more regressed. She refused all communication and we had to feed her. We also had to lift her in and out of bed. But when the music arrived at her bedside, her two feet kept perfect time with the rhythm. Music not only hath charms, it can reach areas that otherwise remain unreachable.

If the patient is ambulatory, dance with him. He will enjoy the one-on-one attention, the physical contact, and the rhythm. We have watched people in Full Care dance, even though their families say they never danced before. I've seen patients put down canes and walkers and enjoy a dance. If the patient is unable to move about the room, let him stand or sit. Hold his hands and gently move them to the rhythm of the music.

Nursing care: Watch for signs of illness

When you are bathing, feeding or doing any other activity with the patient, look for signs of developing physical problems. It is easy to get caught up in a patient's mental problems and overlook a physical problem that might cause odd behavior.

You don't have to do a physical from head to toe, but you should be on the alert for any physical changes. Consult a doctor if any are noted. A few to watch for:

-- Eyes can show dramatic changes with physical illness.

-- Examine the skin for any swelling, changes of color or texture, and/or open or tender areas.

-- Does the patient have guarded movements that might suggest pain?

-- Routinely check the urine and stool for color, blood, frequency and other deviations from normal.

-- Excessive thirst can be a symptom of an illness.

-- Has the patient developed muscle tremors, or are muscles flaccid?

You'll find it much easier to reach a patient on a twin bed instead of a queen or double. Even more preferable is a hospital bed that can be adjusted up and down. This allows the caregiver to lift and turn the patient with less difficulty and without bending. Side rails can help prevent falls.

Nursing care: skin care and bathing

Skin care is of utmost importance, and cleanliness is essential. Sometimes this is difficult to achieve due to the patient's physical as well as mental problems. Often, the patient is unable or unwilling to cooperate.

A routine is usually accepted by the patient and is convenient for the caregiver. The patient should have a bath daily or a shower. If the patient is unable to stand for any length of time, use a shower chair with an open bottom. You can reach all parts of the patient's body if you use a movable hose attached to the shower head.

Keep the patient's hair trimmed in a short, easily-fixed style, to minimize washing and drying times.

If you are unable to get the patient into a tub or shower, you will have to give him a bed bath. Protect the bed from water. Have the patient lie prone, and cover him with a towel or small blanket. Starting with his face, do one part of the body at a time. Turn the patient on one side, and then the other. When you are through, get the patient into a chair and make the bed with clean linens. Try not to let two skin surfaces rub on each other. This is often a source of irritation. You can use a small pillow or folded soft piece of material to do this.

There are many effective moisture barrier creams and lotions on the market to protect the skin from irritation. Your doctor will tell you which one to use.

There are dry shampoos on the market, but none equal a good wash with shampoo and water. It is possible for two people to give the patient a wet shampoo while he is in bed. One holds the patient's head over the edge of the bed; the other washes and rinses the hair with basins and pitchers of water. It's cumbersome, but well worth the trouble.

An important part of skin care is lubrication. After the bath, apply lotion all over the body, giving special attention to bony prominence. Elbows, knees, feet, hips, back and buttocks should get a gentle massage. This not only increases circulation to the area while you are lubricating the skin, it also prevents bed sores.

Bed sores are open areas of the skin caused by pressure and friction of the body against the bedding. Bed sores also are caused by lack of motion, which decreases circulation to the area, and can be aggravated by body excretions left on the skin. These cause irritation and have germs that can cause infection. Small pillows placed under arms, feet, legs, shoulders and other bony areas will change pressure points and help prevent bed sores.

Nursing care: moving the patient

It's important to move a chair-bound patient every hour or two. You don't have to go to a lot of trouble to do this. Stand your loved one up for a minute, rearrange a pillow under him and sit him down again. This will change the pressure on body areas enough to serve your purpose. For added comfort, place pillows under and behind the patient's back. Gently massage pressure areas to aid circulation.

Bed-bound patients need to be moved with the same frequency. This is a little more difficult to do, but it is possible for one person to do it successfully. Fold a twin size sheet in quarters. Place the folded sheet in the center of a bed that is already made. If the patient is in the bed, roll him into it. Otherwise, lay him onto it so that the sheet reaches from head to buttocks. Now you can move the patient by pulling the sheet. Be sure the patient is protected so he cannot roll out of bed while you do this.

To have the patient lie on one side, lift the sheet and slide a pillow in against his back. When it is time to move him again, do the same on the other side, and you have turned the patient with a minimum of time and effort. You might also place small pillows between the legs and under the arms and/or shoulders for added comfort.

It is important to discuss with the doctor whether to keep the patient in bed or to try to get him up and into a chair. Most doctors seem to prefer that the patient be out of bed rather than kept in bed. One person can do this by helping the patient stand, and pivoting him into the chair, but it's best to have help when trying to lift a bed-bound patient into a chair.

A caregiver should never attempt to lift a patient out of a bed or out of a chair unless a physiotherapist or other trained professional has shown the safest method for doing so.

Nursing care: bladder and bowel concerns

Your loved one is confused and is unable to exercise good judgment. This, combined with poor short-term memory, leads to bladder and bowel problems.

The patient knows his bladder area is bothering him, but he may have forgotten that if he passes urine the bladder area will feel better. Or he may have forgotten where the bathroom is. This is hard to believe, but that's what the disease does to people.

Patients don't want to soil themselves. Sometimes they hold the urine until the bladder has a spasm, expels the urine, and causes an "accident." It really isn't an accident, of course. It's perfectly normal for a full bladder to do this.

When such spasms happen repeatedly over a period of time, bladder muscles lose tone and all the urine will not be expelled at one void. Compare this to a balloon that never goes back to its original size after it has been blown up. Incomplete voiding of urine can lead to a bladder infection. To prevent this, routinely take your loved one to the bathroom every two to three hours. When you do this, be sure he wipes, flushes and washes. He will need to be reminded.

Bowel problems also are common in Alzheimer's disease patients. They may forget how to push the stool out of the rectum, or a lack of coordination may make it difficult for them to push. The result is a bowel impaction or an involuntary evacuation. Naturally you want to avoid this if at all possible.

Once again, it's important to establish a routine. Take the patient to the bathroom at the same time every day. After breakfast is usually the best time for most people. Once this routine is established, it almost becomes a conditioned reflex to expel the stool.

Diet and fluids play an important role in having a successful bowel evacuation. Bowel function is directly related to good nutrition and well being. Perhaps the most common problem is constipation. The patient's poor muscle control prevents him from coordinating enough to empty the bowel, and the stool in the rectum hardens.

Adequate fluids and roughage, coupled with timing to create a conditioned reflex, usually solve the problem. Once again I refer you to the patient's doctor for advice if this is inadequate.

Partial adult diapers are a help for a patient who loses a little urine or stool infrequently. He will feel more secure and avoid embarrassment. Partial diapers also have elastic on the sides, which make it easy for the patient to pull them up and down without assistance.

Full-size adult diapers can be wonderful for people who frequently are incontinent of urine or involuntary of stool, but many patients find the full diaper clumsy to pull up and down.

Always keep a watchful eye on the patient when he uses the bathroom. He may be confused and poorly coordinated, yet will feel embarrassed if he finds himself soiled. Patients often don't know what to do with diapers, and may hide them, or even put them in their pockets.

They also may use the laundry hamper, closets or any other available place instead of the toilet. So go into the bathroom with your patient. Expect some protest when you start to do this. Simply say, "I have to be here," and/or give some privacy by turning your back. Patients usually get used to the idea and will accept the caregiver's presence.

Be sure to wear rubber gloves if it is necessary to come in contact with the patient's body fluids.

If your loved one is bed-bound, you might want to ask the doctor about a tube called a Foley catheter. When placed (by a medical professional) into the bladder through the urethra, it drains the urine into a plastic bag. But there can be side effects; be sure to discuss this possibility with the doctor.

Nursing care: other hygiene concerns

Fingernails need special attention. They grow too long, break, get dirty and often become unsightly. A few minutes soak in a small bowl of soap and warm water, followed by a gentle brushing should keep them clean. Use a nail clip or file as needed to keep the hands manicured.

Toenails need special attention, too. They should be cut straight across. Be on the alert for ingrown toenails. These often are caused by tight socks, shoes or pressure from bedclothes. A podiatrist should see any infections of the feet.

Check eye glasses and hearing aids from time to time for comfort of fit and effectiveness. Hearing aid batteries wear out and should be replaced; accumulated dirt should be cleaned.

Mouth care is of utmost importance, and brushing after meals can be a comfort to the patient. Dentures or bridges should be cared for after meals because food can get under them, which can be annoying to the patient. Be sure to check for dental problems or ill fitting dentures.

Ill fitting dentures or teeth that are painful are often the cause of poor appetite. The patient is unable to tell you that the teeth or dentures are hurting, and because of the discomfort, he refuses to eat.

There is a trick to removing dentures from a patient who is unable to do it for himself. Tell the patient ahead of time what you plan to do. I usually say, "I'm going to clean your teeth and give them right back to you. You will feel better after I do that." Seldom do I get any objections.

Wet your index finger with water and slide your finger along the top edge of the denture. When you get to the tooth before the last one, place your finger on the top of the denture and press down gently. This breaks the vacuum and allows the denture to fall loose.

Nursing care: food and nutrition

Unfortunately, when the illness progresses to this point, the loved one is usually losing weight and the caregiver is having difficulty getting him to eat and drink.

The patient's reflexes are diminished and his incentive to eat is low. He is lethargic and busy with hallucinations. Food does not interest him. Yet food and fluid intake are important to his well being.

Many patients have difficulty chewing and swallowing, and choking is not uncommon. They have difficulty using a knife, fork and spoon properly. A patient will put food on a spoon and then lose it on the way to his mouth.

You will find yourself helping your patient or feeding him most of the time. Be certain he does not pocket the food in his cheek instead of swallowing the food. Sometimes patients end up with a mouthful of food that is impossible to swallow.

There are so many special diets and fads today that I find it difficult to recommend or dispute any of them. My feeling is that too much of a good thing is not good. I advise you to stay away from all fads. Your goal is to provide your loved one with good food in moderation.

Alzheimer's patients often don't eat properly due to the confusion seen throughout the disease. Vitamin and mineral supplements may be needed. The patient's doctor is the one who should govern these additions to the diet.

Also consult the doctor if you notice any change in the patient's appetite. There are medical problems not related to Alzheimer's that can increase or decrease appetite. Digestive problems can effect the appetite, for example, and the patient would be unable to describe any symptoms to his caregiver.

Sometimes a patient's taste changes and he will want sweet things. That's OK. Once again your imagination and ingenuity come into play. Do whatever works to induce your patient to eat wholesome food, even if it means mixing ice cream into the meat or vegetables. Sounds terrible, doesn't it? It works. I use Jell-O and chocolate pudding a lot, with great success most of the time.

Difficulty in chewing is common. If you have already ruled out any problems with teeth or dentures, then you have to suspect the patient's coordination. Just as he is losing coordination in his arms and legs, he is losing coordination with activities such as chewing. It's just not as noticeable.

You may find your patient spitting food out, refusing food, pocketing it in his cheeks and/or putting food in his hand. He is unable to tell you something is wrong, and this may be his way of responding to his inability to chew properly.

It may help to cut the food into small pieces, as we discussed in Partial Care, or puree his food. If he chokes easily on liquids, pureed food may be easier to swallow. It seems to stimulate the swallow reflex better than liquids. Test it with small spoonfuls if your doctor thinks it is advisable.

You can puree meat, carrots, celery and many other good foods. You might combine two or more good foods to make a semi-liquid, like mixing milk with mashed potatoes. If meat is dry and sticks in the patient's mouth, mix something with a soft, smooth texture (like pureed carrots or peaches) in with it. Do whatever helps the food slide down with less effort.

Choking happens because the patient's reflexes are diminished. The epiglottis, which covers the windpipe when he swallows, often does not close in time and the food enters the windpipe. This seriously interferes with breathing, and is an immediate concern.

To minimize the danger of choking, provide food cut into small pieces and watch that the patient does not put too much food into his mouth at one time. Consider the texture of the food. Give a little bit of food at a time instead of the entire meal. Be certain they eat slowly.

If you notice the patient having trouble chewing or swallowing, remove the food completely. It is better to miss a meal than to choke. Tell your doctor about the feeding problem and ask him to advise you the best route to follow.

Hallucinations also can be a deterrent to eating. The patient becomes so busy with seeing and hearing things that are not there that he forgets the real world. As we mentioned in Partial Care, you often can break a hallucination with a question or a statement. If this doesn't work, take the patient's face gently between your hands, look into his eyes and talk to him.

You will also have to deal with the patient's forgetfulness. For example, he may have a glass of juice on the table in front of him, and he would like to drink the juice. However, he has forgotten how. It may sound incredible, but this can happen.

Deal with this by saying quietly, "Take a drink of juice," as you put the glass in his hand and bring it to his mouth. This will likely trigger a conditioned reflex and he will follow through by drinking. Incidentally, it is better if the patient pours liquid into his own mouth rather than if you do if for him. The hand-to-mouth movement will place the head back, into a better position for swallowing.

Caregivers should watch for signs of dehydration (infrequent urination, dry mouth, sunken eyes, wrinkled skin that lacks elasticity). People need fluids in all kinds of weather, and warm weather demands more fluids. It is always easier to prevent a problem than to treat it after it occurs, so take time to stay with your loved one while he is drinking to make sure he takes in enough fluid.

Snacks between meals are an excellent way to get more food and fluids into a sick person. Patients seem to fill up quickly at meal time and are eager for snacks.

You can make snacks from wholesome foods with no extra effort.

A caregiver's checklist for Stage Five
   -- Do not attempt Full Care without assistance.
   -- Exercise the patient by moving each part of the body gently.
   -- Allow children and pets to play with the patient.
   -- Take the patient outdoors several times a day.
   -- Give the patient pleasure with music.
   -- Dance with him, or move his arms gently to the music.
   -- Be on the alert for signs of developing physical problems.
   -- Provide the patient with a twin bed or hospital bed.
   -- Bathe the patient daily, and give a bed bath if necessary.
   -- Keep the patient's hair short for easy care.
   -- Lubricate and massage the skin to prevent bed sores.
   -- Cushion sensitive areas of the body with pillows.
   -- Move a chair- or bed-bound patient every hour or two.
   -- Discuss with the patient's doctor whether the patient should be kept in bed, and concerning the use of a catheter.
   -- Always have assistance when trying to lift the patient (or ask a physiotherapist how to do it safely by yourself).
   -- Establish a routine to avoid bladder and bowel problems.
   -- Wear rubber gloves if you must come in contact with body fluids.

-- Provide partial adult diapers or full diapers as needed.

-- Always accompany the patient when he goes to the bathroom.

-- Keep fingernails and toenails clean and trimmed.

-- Watch for dental problems, clean the patient's dentures and/or assist the patient in brushing after meals.

-- Check glasses and hearing aids for cleanliness, fit and effectiveness.

-- Use your imagination and ingenuity to induce the patient to eat wholesome food.

-- Provide food that can be eaten with minimal effort.

-- Take precautions to avoid choking.

-- Watch for signs of dehydration.

-- Provide frequent snacks to ensure adequate fluids and nourishment.

Chapter Nine

Placement Outside the Home

Before you consider placing your loved one permanently in a skilled care facility, you might want to try temporary respite care out of the home. As we mentioned in Chapter Two, there are facilities that will care for your patient on a short-term basis. This not only gives you a respite, but is a good test of how well your loved one will react to being outside the home, and to being cared for by a trained staff.

You might try temporary respite care for a long weekend. This will give you a change of pace, and a chance to get a good rest physically and mentally, and to have some fun.

If all goes well, you might want to use temporary respite care later on for a week or two. Take a vacation, give yourself a total change of environment, perhaps visit friends or relatives. You will come back refreshed and better able to continue your task of giving your loved one the best care possible. You also will have restored your positive attitude and sense of humor. The experience will be good for all concerned.

A word of caution, when leaving a loved one in a skilled care facility: It is difficult for the staff to keep track of clothing and valuables. All clothing should be marked clearly with the patient's name. Any valuable papers, cards or jewelry should be kept at home or replaced with unimportant or inexpensive substitutes.

Be certain your loved one wears his identification bracelet at all times. If by chance he should wander, this is crucial.

Have a dentist label the patient's dentures. I have seen patients take dentures out and put them on their dinner plates, and then the dentures get a ride to the kitchen. Patients will also put their dentures under their pillows, and then the dentures are bundled up with the laundry. When they turn up in the kitchen or the laundry, it's hard for such items to be identified and returned to their proper owners.

Glasses also should be labeled. When I worked in a resident facility, I found a sweet little lady in a wheel chair with six pairs of glasses in her lap. She had gone room to room and picked up glasses. Why? No answer to that. She didn't touch anything else, and she willingly gave them to me. Incidentally, she was wearing her own glasses at the time. As you might imagine, we had a terrible time finding out who each pair belonged to.

Fortunately, at most facilities, the staff is trained to watch for such things. But they can't be everywhere at once.

Making a difficult decision

You may become very upset once you come to the full realization that you are no longer able to care for your loved one at home. Even though you have known since the early onset of the disease that this time would come, you never wanted to see the day.

As the overburdened caregiver, the decision is yours. I wish some magic could take the decision from you and eliminate your grief.

Once again I urge you to make an effort to be objective. Make a list of pros and cons, discuss it with friends and relatives, and speak with the patient's doctor. Talk about it at your support group.

Above all, don't allow yourself to feel guilty. You have done the best you are able to do up to this point, and if you cannot extend yourself any further, the time has come to place your loved one outside the home.

Remember, earlier in the book, we said to take care of the caregiver. We can't let you get sick, and that's what will happen if you are overextended for a long period of time. Again, everyone has a different capacity, so don't compare yourself to anyone else. Assess your own particular situation.

Usually by this time caregivers are tired and frustrated. The patient is irrational and requires constant management. Neither patient nor caregiver gets a good night's sleep. The situation escalates and becomes unacceptable for all concerned.

You have been through a long, tough ordeal and it isn't over yet. You and your loved one are entering a new phase of this disaster that has happened to you. Have courage. You are not alone. There are many people who understand what you are going through, so use them as your support.

Evaluating skilled care facilities

You will want to visit as many skilled care facilities as possible, preferably those that specializes in Alzheimer's disease. Talk to the staff, look at the patients and evaluate the surroundings. Here is a checklist that may help:

-- Does the staff seem interested, kind and knowledgeable?

-- Do the patients seem content?

-- Do the patients look clean and neat?

110 -- Eileen Driscoll

-- Is the facility clean? Is there an odor of urine?
-- Are the day rooms comfortable?
-- Is the facility locked securely?
-- Is the food good and served in a pleasant manner?
-- What are the sleeping arrangements?
-- Is it crowded or is there ample room to move about?
-- Are there planned activities for those who can participate?

Talk to people in your support group who have a direct knowledge of the facility. Also, research your options. One paperback book that covers this subject in detail is "Choosing a Nursing Home," by Seth Goldsmith, Ph.D., published by Prentice Hall Press (1990).

Keep in mind that placement is not final. If you choose a facility and it does not give your loved one the care you desire, you can move him elsewhere. It is better to avoid such a move, but sometimes it happens. Follow your own good judgment and do what you feel is right.

Dealing with depression

Once your loved one has been placed outside the home you will feel a void that may be, at times, over-whelming.

After all, you have been working at a steady pace with no relief for a long time. Your loved one is no longer with you and all of a sudden you find you have nothing to do.

Expect to feel depressed. You may also feel guilty, as though you have abandoned your loved one. These feelings are normal, but you can't allow them to govern your life. You and only you can change the picture you are looking at now.

Fill the void with something you enjoy doing. There are many activities to choose from. You may not feel like doing anything in the beginning, but you should make yourself do something. Try to keep busy. Volunteer work is one solution. Work with children instead of adults for a change of pace.

Try to find a happy, upbeat environment. You might take up bridge or go on outings with friends or neighborhood groups. Once you know your loved one is settled comfortably you can take a little vacation.

Visit your loved one frequently. The patient has learned that his primary caregiver is the one he depends on and looks to for security, even though he no longer knows if the caregiver is a wife, daughter, husband or any other relationship. Your frequent visits will reassure your loved one he still has a familiar source of security as he adjusts to the staff of the facility. This can be traumatic for the patient but it is essential for him and his caregiver.

If you need to, allow yourself a time to cry. Give yourself ten or 15 minutes to let out all your frustration, anger, grief or anything else that is upsetting you. Then go and do something good for yourself.

I think it is normal to feel depressed at a time like this. Don't chastise yourself for it. The disease you have had to deal with created a drastic change in your life, and it was nothing but trouble. Be careful not to dwell on your depression. Allow it to come out briefly, then make a conscious effort to place your thoughts on pleasant things.

I'd like to share an experience with you that, though not exactly what you are going through, is similar.

My husband died when I was 55 years old. After he died, I lay awake for three nights without sleeping.

During the day I walked about the house, doing nothing but feeling sorry for myself. Finally I sat myself down and had a good talk. I came to the conclusion that I could either continue as I had been and destroy myself, or I could fashion a new life for myself.

This was over ten years ago and I still miss my husband. Yet I have also gone onto new things and enjoy them. Life changes, and you have to allow the changes or you will remain very unhappy. It isn't easy. You have to work hard at it sometimes, but that's the healthy way to deal with a problem such as this.

It helps to remember that your life would not have been as rich without that beloved spouse, parent or friend. Some people go through life and never experience the true love relationship you had with your loved one for so many years. Really, those who grieve for a loved one, whether ill or deceased, are the lucky ones. They have experienced such wonderful love in their lives.

Many people find church groups to be a big help. As I said before, God has His reasons and we often don't know why. You may not like this, but that's the way it is, and you have no choice but to deal with it.

Look ahead to a brighter future

I have another story for you that illustrates how to cope with a difficult time in your life. I do not recommend that you follow my exact footsteps, only that you allow yourself to be open to creative and unusual ways of dealing with your depression and grief.

I once was faced with a problem I couldn't change, and I was forced to cope with it for an extended period of time. I continually asked myself, "What am I going to do?" It was on my mind day and night and nothing seemed to erase it for me.

Believe it or not, I solved my problem by going to Clown School, something that had always intrigued me. I became a clown and joined Clown Alley. This may seem like a crazy way to cope with a problem, yet it worked.

First I was busy deciding what kind of a clown I wanted to be. Next, original make-up had to be designed. Then I needed a clown name, and I chose Merrily. I also had to make a costume. During this process I met a wonderful group of people. After class we would go to an ice cream parlor for sundaes and sodas and blow up balloons for all the kids who were there. Several of us worked out skits to do in schools.

We loved each other and what we were doing. We went to parades, schools, nursing homes, meetings for the deaf and many other places together. The clowns were my answer, and my problem has since resolved itself. I often think that if that particular problem had never presented itself, I never would have found the camaraderie and friendship I experienced with that clown group.

No doubt becoming a clown is be the farthest thing from your mind. Yet there is, without doubt, something very special waiting for you, and I urge you to look for it. When one door closes, another seems to open for us.

And when you find your special activity or vocation, I hope it will lighten your burden, bring out the best in you, give joy to others, and provide you with wonderful new friends. You certainly deserve all these things.

Chapter Ten
An Alzheimer's Case History

To help you better understand the progress of Alzheimer's disease from beginning to end, I am going to give you a hypothetical case history. The names and places are fictitious.

The caregiver and family in the following case history pretty much do everything right. I felt it would be more helpful to give an uplifting example, rather than to mention all the mistakes caregivers and families can make.

Mary is the patient. Her husband and primary caregiver is John. Their children are Joe, Bob and Ann. Mary was diagnosed in 1982, when she and her husband were both 66 years old. Mary had Alzheimer's disease for ten years prior to her death in 1992.

Before the disease

Mary and John grew up in Wisconsin and met in college. Soon after graduation, in 1938, they were married. Mary became a teacher, specialized in the sciences, and became the head of the science department of the high school where she taught. She was proud of the number of students she was able to send to college on science scholarships.

John used his business background to start a motel and restaurant on a lake shore in Minnesota. They had a thriving business after just a few years.

Over the next ten years, Mary and John had two sons and one daughter. Mary stopped working, stayed at home and was content as a housewife and mother.

When the children were in high school, Mary started helping John in the motel. She busied herself in the restaurant section and was able to increase the profits with good planning, buying and decorating. She added new recipes to enhance the menu. John took care of the motel's repairs and upkeep, billing and other chores. The money they saved by having Mary work in the restaurant helped defray some of the children's college expenses.

After graduation, their oldest child, Joe, found employment in California with an aircraft manufacturing company. Joe married and had three children.

Second son Bob became a TV producer and worked in New York. Bob and his wife had two children.

Ann married a hometown boy, had three children and lived about 25 miles from her parents. In all, Mary and John had eight grandchildren.

Joe and Bob came to visit on holidays and vacations, bringing their families with them. Ann visited more often because she and her family lived closer.

Mary is diagnosed

One day, when she was 66 years old, Mary went to lunch with some ladies from her club. John became concerned when Mary was not home in time for supper. When Mary did come home, she was upset, and said there had been a detour and she got lost. John accepted this.

Soon after, there were no eggs in stock to cook breakfast for the motel guests. Mary had forgotten to order them. John was able to buy some quickly and the problem was solved.

On another occasion, Mary told John to call Joe because his wife was sick. It turned out it was Bob's son, and he had been in a car accident. Mary couldn't understand how the story got so mixed up, and was angry with John for not calling the right son.

There were other small incidents similar to these, and John began to think something was wrong with Mary. Maybe her blood pressure? John noticed Mary had been unusually disorganized. He spoke with Ann about it and they agreed Mary should see a doctor. Mary was reluctant to go but went after much coaxing. John was truly concerned about Mary.

The family doctor was very understanding and also very thorough. He did many tests on Mary because he had to rule out a number of neurological diseases, some that are easily treated, and others that are not. He also had to rule out systemic diseases that can cause neuro-logical problems. The tests came back negative. His diagnosis was Alzheimer's disease.

The doctor explained to the family that there was no test for Alzheimer's. He had made the diagnosis by ruling out other possible causes of the symptoms Mary was presenting.

The diagnosis frightened the entire family. Ann's first concern was for her mother's future. Then she wondered if she too might develop Alzheimer's in the future.

John was upset, realizing his wife would no longer be responsible for the household, the restaurant, or for that matter, anything else.

Mary also was upset because she knew something was wrong. She tried to cover her mistakes and was ashamed to talk about it with anyone.

Ann called her brothers and told them what the doctor had said. Both flew home so they could have a family get-together and make plans for the future.

Fortunately, the family had an excellent and understanding M.D. He explained the disease to them and gave them literature to read. He also suggested they get more information from the library and from the Alzheimer's Association.

They soon realized the magnitude of the problem they were facing. The doctor assured Ann that there was no proof that the disease is inherited. He also advised the family to seek legal advice.

They consulted the law firm that John used for the motel and other incidental legal matters. The attorney suggested that they sell their business since they were both 66 years of age, ready for retirement and had saved a good nest egg for their old age.

John sold the motel and restaurant, bought a smaller home in the same area, and invested the income from the sale. The attorney took steps to protect their assets as prudently as possible. Mary adjusted well to the move.

Mary loved and trusted her family and appreciated how wonderfully they treated her. She partially understood her illness. She was aware of the fact that she was making mistakes yet could not understand why, even though the doctor explained it to her.

She had no idea her judgment was impaired, and she never did understand this. John reassured her repeatedly that he would help her, but she cried almost every day. Mary found that she could not make John understand what she was trying to tell him. She didn't realize she was substituting incorrect words or that her conversation didn't make sense at times. She just knew something was wrong, and it upset her.

Early stages of the disease: Aware and Acceptance

Mary began to vacillate from Stage One, Aware to Stage Two, Acceptance daily. She was aware of her illness and accepted as much as she was able.

Let's look at what was happening to Mary.

In Mary's brain, the tangles had started slowly, even before she got lost on the way home. They affected her ability to reach the area of her brain that allowed her to remember the route home. Yet they had not affected the area of the brain that allowed her to recognize the fact that she was lost and confused, and this frightened her.

She already had been aware of other things that were not quite right, but this was the first big thing that she couldn't deny by simply saying, "I made a mistake," or, "I forgot."

At first she denied that anything was really wrong. Then she felt anger, "Why is this happening to me?" And then she felt ashamed, and tried to hide her errors. When she was diagnosed, she felt exposed, and was even more ashamed and angry.

She even thought, "Maybe this is someone else's fault. They are playing tricks on me." Her reasoning and information processing systems were slightly affected. This was a terrible time for Mary. She was hurting badly because she knew she was making mistakes, and was unable to prevent them.

Now let's take a look at what was happening to John, other family members and their friends during the same time.

John loved his wife dearly. He and Mary and their children had always been a close-knit family. When John and the children held the family meeting at the onset of Mary's illness, they agreed that John would be her primary caregiver. They also agreed to help as much as possible, and felt secure with this decision.

They read a great deal to further their understanding of Alzheimer's disease, to plan for the future, and to give Mary the best care. They also decided to keep Mary at home for as long as possible, rather than in a skilled nursing facility. They learned not to expect anything from Mary, and saw whatever she was able to do as a bonus for all of them.

Her family excused Mary's behavior 100 percent of the time. They made a point of having fun together and agreed not to let the illness stop them from enjoying her company, or each other's. They agreed that the grand-children would also be included as much as possible in Mary's care.

When John and Ann attended an Alzheimer's support group in their area they felt relieved. They were able to share their distress and fears with other people who totally understood, because they were experiencing the same crisis. John and Ann also decided to enlist any help available to them among friends and family, for long term care and for respite.

John and Mary had cultivated a small circle of good friends and also had brothers and sisters in the area. John spoke to all of them privately and told them what the doctor had said about Mary's illness. John request-ed that they keep contact and continue their friendship.

He also asked them if they might possibly stay with Mary occasionally as a respite for him.

They maintained their friendship with a few special friends and these people were like gold to John. Others among their group of friends stopped inviting them for meetings, dinner or cards, and John felt this acutely. John allowed them to remove themselves, assuming a lack of understanding or embarrassment when Mary made a "mistake."

John and Mary's brothers and sisters reacted in ways similar to the friends. Some continued to share in the family's get-togethers; others were "too busy to come." Again John accepted this gracefully even though it hurt him deeply.

Mary was still able to cook dinner with a little help from John, and she enjoyed going out to dinner too. They appreciated the company of those who came to visit them more than ever.

The ways that Alzheimer's disease affects a caregiver and family began to impact John.

He was unable to rely on Mary for important things that needed to be done, and did them himself.

He had to make sure Mary was safe at all times.

He had to watch her to be sure she didn't turn the stove on and forget about it.

He was unable to rely on her for telephone messages.

He was the only one with a car in the family.

He lost friends he had thought were good friends.

He was virtually estranged from some relatives on both sides of the family.

He had to take care of the finances without assistance.

He felt lonely at times, even though he had good family support and good friends.

He felt totally frustrated knowing there was no medicine that could help.

He felt afraid of what the future might bring in terms of Mary's illness.

Even with all the help that was offered and available, John still felt overwhelmed. He realized he would have to rely strongly on his ability to adapt.

John was also a deeply religious man. He leaned on his faith in God to see him through hard times. John reflected on the long, happy marriage he and Mary had, and the wonderful family they had raised. These thoughts helped him greatly.

He would give Mary hugs, and she always hugged back. This gave him the courage to continue the hard job before him. No, he told himself, it wouldn't be easy. But he would take care of his wonderful wife when she was unable to take care of herself, and he would do it graciously and willingly.

He often thought about people less fortunate than himself who never had good marriages or close families, and he knew their lives were much worse than his. Even so, he did feel overwhelmed at times.

John also decided to make the most of a bad situation. He decided he and Mary would enjoy as much as she was able before her illness destroyed parts of the brain that still were functioning. He evaluated her situation realistically and decided there was still time to have fun together. They would take it one day at a time.

Hopefully, Mary had reached a plateau, and the illness would progress slowly enough to allow them more good time together. They would go on a vacation and visit friends and family in other states.

John made plans to stay in Wisconsin and have an old fashioned holiday season with family and friends. They had done this often during the years before Mary became ill. He then made plans to fly to California to visit Joe and his family, and, in the spring, to visit New York City and stay with Bob and his family.

John proceeded to outline a few other visits and was happy with the plans. Mary was excited about their travel plans, too. 1983 and 1984 were good years for them. They traveled, and also were home some of the time.

Mary is Unaware, and requires Partial Care

However, the terrible things that were happening in Mary's brain continued their work of destruction. John knew Mary was becoming sicker. Mary became less aware of errors and leaned on him more and more.

Her conversation was hesitant. She had difficulty completing a sentence and would lose her thought midway in a story. She often used incorrect words and could not find a word she wanted to use. Before long, John had to do all the shopping and cooking.

Mary would forget where the bathroom was and John would have to show her. Sometimes she forgot to flush. He also had to assist Mary whenever she took a shower. She wouldn't dry herself or couldn't find the clothes he left out for her. Sometimes she couldn't get her clothes on by herself, and he would help.

When they noticed Mary having difficulty dressing, Ann and John took her shopping and bought clothes that were easy to take on and off. They bought slacks that had elastic waist bands instead of zippers, buttons or belts. They found shoes with Velcro closing instead of laces and substituted low heel slip-on shoes for those with higher heels, because Mary's coordination was not as good as it used to be. They also bought loose-fitting, slip-on blouses and sweaters.

Next, they took Mary to the beauty parlor and had her hair done in an easy-care style that was attractive. They had anticipated doing all of this. It was all part of the planning the family had done shortly after Mary was diagnosed.

Several times Mary had an accident and wet her pants. After that, John saw to it Mary was reminded to go to the bathroom at timely intervals. If they were going to be gone from home for several hours, John would see that Mary had an adult diaper in place. This was just in case Mary didn't get to the bathroom in time. It made things easier for all concerned, prevented problems and avoided embarrassment.

Mary wandered about the house frequently, touching or picking up things for no reason. When this habit started, John would leave out towels that needed folding or handkerchiefs or socks to be matched from the laundry. This would often occupy Mary for long periods of time and gave John a chance to work or rest peacefully.

About the same time, John removed all the valuable figurines and glassware from the house and packed them away safely so Mary would not break them accidentally. He did this for her, now that she was unable to do it herself. John knew Mary had planned to save the good pieces for their children and grandchildren.

He replaced the items with attractive, inexpensive things that were not breakable. Mary could pick up and drop anything she wanted to, and no harm would be done.

Once, while John was speaking on the telephone, Mary wandered out of the house. A neighbor saw her and brought her home. This was traumatic for John. Mary was unaware of what had happened. John installed sound alarms on all the doors to the house, so he would know his wife was safely in the house at all times.

At the same time, he had a lock put on his workshop to protect Mary from his power tools and other sharp objects.

Mary had been ill for the past four years and was regressing rapidly.

She was usually quiet and pleasant, but there was now almost no conversation between them. Much of the time Mary was unable to understand what was said, and was also unable to answer.

This particularly depressed John. He felt very alone. In essence, his wife was gone. She was there physically, but her "self or her brain" was no longer functioning the way it once did. Their sex life was over. She still responded to his hug or kiss but was unable to respond in an intimate relationship.

They no longer could have fun together, yet Mary still had the capacity to experience some feelings. She always knew if she was happy or sad, and he knew it was important to keep her happy.

John still loved her dearly and intended to keep his promise of caring for her as well as he was able, but he felt himself becoming angry and frustrated almost daily. He was tired. He had no time for himself. John knew he needed time away from Mary at this point in her illness, and Ann tried to help him as much as possible.

John decided to establish a routine that would provide good care for Mary, and that would also give him time with friends or to be alone. It would also allow him time to do the household chores with fewer problems.

Mary was confused most of the time, and sometimes did not even recognize John. He decided to do all the necessary things himself and allow Mary to do whatever she was able to do.

In the morning after breakfast, John and Mary got into the shower together. This was easier for John, rather than trying to stay dry while helping Mary. He laid out all the towels and clothes ahead of time.

Once they were both dressed John made breakfast. Sometimes Mary did the dishes but most of the time she just sat and watched John. After breakfast they walked for about a mile around the neighborhood.

John arranged respite with two couples, also retired, who volunteered their time. One couple were long-time friends; the other were Mary's sister and her husband. Each couple came once a week. The men would play golf while the ladies stayed with Mary and did some sewing or a simple craft with her. The men ate lunch out, and the conversation with other men was a treat for John.

One evening a week they alternated going to each other's homes. They played cards or a game, had snacks and enjoyed each other's company. Mary couldn't take part in the games or cards but she sat at the table with them and understood some of the conversation. They all felt comfortable with this arrangement.

On Sundays, John and Mary attended church. Afterwards, twice a month, they would go to Ann's house for the day. Mary loved her three grandchildren.

She enjoyed watching them play and they interacted well with her. On these Sundays, Mary would stay overnight, and this gave John the following Monday to do the heavy cleaning and shopping without having to keep an eye on her.

Ann would take her mother and children to the park and bring Mary home in the late afternoon. If it was raining they would play a game at home or do a craft of some sort. The children were wonderful with Mary. They would help her with her craft or show her how to paint, and they all seemed to enjoy each other. There were a lot of smiles and hugs and some good laughs too.

Sometimes Mary and the grandchildren all took a nap together. They would all snuggle up in the big bed and drift off to sleep for an hour. This gave Ann some quiet time to herself.

Little by little, physical changes in Mary became obvious. Her balance was poor. She walked with a hesitant, wide stride. She tripped often and fell several times. She wasn't always sure which direction she was going. She couldn't find the kitchen.

Sometimes she would go to sit on a chair and almost miss it. If John gave Mary a book and asked her to put it on the table she would walk around the room, evidently unable to find the table. The area of Mary's brain that governed spatial perception had been affected by the illness.

Mary had difficulty knowing where she was in relation to other things in the room. Since she was presenting more new problems frequently, it was becoming more difficult for John's volunteer helpers to care for Mary.

John and Ann attended their support group weekly whenever possible. When Bob and Joe and their families came to visit, they also attended. They found it helped to share their problem with others who could empathize, and who also could offer advice.

Members of the support group suggested day care to Ann and John several times before they decided to test it out. John had mixed emotions. He knew the staff would take good care of Mary. He had observed the day care center whenever he attended support group meetings in the same building. Other caregivers had their loved ones in the day care, and had given him positive feedback.

Yet placing her in day care felt to John as though he was, to some extent, abandoning Mary. He also was afraid of upsetting her more than necessary. And how could he give his precious Mary to strangers for a whole day? Mary didn't know any of them and would be afraid. Besides, hadn't he promised to take care of her himself? His conscience bothered him. He felt like a traitor.

These and other questions plagued John. What would happen if Mary had an accident and wet herself? Would they understand the way he did? Suppose Mary got agitated and pushed them away, as she did with him occasionally? What if Mary didn't like it there?

Finally John realized he was looking at his problem subjectively instead of objectively. He knew he was getting good advice from the support group. He realized he was worn out physically and mentally from constant daily caregiving. He also knew he needed more respite for himself if he was going to continue to care for Mary over the long term.

Friends in the support group also told him that their loved ones had done well in day care. They felt the planned activities and socialization kept some patients' social skills functioning, even better than when they were home with just their caregivers. He also heard that patients enjoyed the day care program.

John decided to test day care for Mary, and Ann agreed it was a good idea. Since the staff specialized in the care of Alzheimer's patients, it certainly seemed a safe place to leave Mary, and one that might even produce positive results.

Mary's first day in day care was very difficult. She was frightened, cried and responded poorly to the staff and the other patients. She refused to join any activities, wandered and looked out the windows and doors constantly.

John was upset, too. He knew he was doing the right thing, yet couldn't shake the feeling that he was abandoning his beloved wife. When he returned to the peace and quiet of his home he had time to sit and think objectively. He confirmed his decision to utilize day care for Mary.

John took Mary to day care several times a week. She adjusted to the people and the surroundings in a short period of time. The staff was able to give John favorable reports on Mary's behavior and reactions.

This was a big relief to John. It gave him physical relief from Mary's care and mental relief from the constant watchfulness that was so necessary. More and more, he was feeling the need to be relieved from care problems. As Mary got sicker, John used the day care system more frequently.

He was tired, and he was getting older, too. He was grateful to God for his good health, but knew it was of utmost importance that he stay well. The day care center filled a need in John's life.

Mary was in day care for three years before the ravages of the illness meant another change of plans for John. When Mary began to enter Stage Five, Full Care, she was 73 years old and had been ill for seven years.

Mary requires Full Care

John had trouble understanding how his wife, who had cooked so many delicious meals and set such a beautiful table, could forgot how to use a knife and fork.

Mealtimes were difficult for John. Mary had almost forgotten how to eat. He had to cut her meat and other foods into small pieces, and she would often use her fingers instead of utensils.

Mary was not getting enough to eat and drink. She was slowly losing weight, and the doctor suggested John give her a commercially-prepared fortified drink. This helped to stop the weight loss and maintain her health. Before long, John had to feed Mary most of her meals.

Mary gradually had begun to hallucinate several months earlier. In the beginning this lasted for just a fleeting moment, then, as time went by, the hallucinations lasted longer and became more noticeable. Eventually Mary saw things that were imaginary and did not see what was real, most of the time.

Mary often spoke to the imaginary visions in garbled speech. Sometimes her speech would take on a rhythmic sound and she would rock with its rhythm. In order to get Mary to do something, John would have to work through the hallucination to get her attention.

Mary was now more difficult to care for because she was unable to cooperate with her caregiver. She did not understand that John was trying to change her clothes or feed her. She had no comprehension of what was going on in the world around her.

Mary vacillated between being hyperactive or passive each day. She would walk about the house quickly, with no apparent purpose other than constant movement. She would move chairs, lamps, books and anything else in the room from one place to the other for no reason.

To make matters worse, Mary's coordination was poor and hallucinations prevented her from seeing obstacles in her way or even the chair she was trying to sit in. Mary had several falls and many near falls. When John tried to stop this activity or move her to a safe area of the house, she would strike at him with surprising strength. She would even try to run or pull away from him.

Mary had no idea who John was or where she was. Sometimes after a spell of irrational activity, Mary would sit in a chair and stare into space for long periods of time with no reaction at all. It was as difficult to break this staring pattern as it was to quiet the hyperactivity.

John could no longer leave Mary with volunteer caregivers. They were unable to cope with her behavior, and they too were getting older. Ann tried to help but her growing family limited her time.

Reports from the day care center also were discouraging. Mary was no longer able to take part in activities because she no longer understood anything said to her. Her information processing system had been almost completely destroyed by her illness. Mary had also become disruptive on several occasions. When this happened the day care staff would call John at home and he would go immediately and bring Mary home.

John realized he was getting close to the time when he would no longer be able to care for Mary at home. Her illness was more than one person could handle.

Mary's care took too much time and energy. He constantly felt fatigued, mentally and physically.

John also knew that if anything happened to him there was no one else who could care for Mary at home. He realized, if he was going to exercise good judgment, he had to place Mary in a skilled care facility.

Once again his support group came to his assistance, and provided the names of several facilities in the area. These were accredited by the State Department of Licenses. Some of the members of the support group had already placed their loved ones in skilled care facilities and had good reports for John.

John and Ann visited several facilities, and chose one that had a good reputation and was close to home. When the time came for Mary to be placed in the facility, John and Ann went through the same agonizing doubts and emotions they experienced earlier when leaving Mary at the day care center.

They leaned heavily on each other. John and his daughter both knew they had made the right decision, yet they couldn't help but feel resentful. Why had they been forced to make such a difficult decision? They looked around them and saw many older couples going about their daily lives, apparently at ease and free of problems. John and Ann felt jealous of their happy lifestyles. Why did this terrible thing happen to their wife and mother?

They shared a quiet time together and once again their faith in God helped them. No one knows why one person has an easy life and another person has a difficult life. When John and Ann counted the blessings of years gone by and the blessings they still had, they knew that even with all their trouble they had truly been blessed.

With relaxed minds, knowing they were doing the right thing, they brought Mary to the facility they had chosen. They knew she would be given quality care, and that it would be administered with love by a well-trained staff. They rested in the knowledge that they had done the best possible for Mary in the past, and that this was the best choice under the present circumstances.

Mary did not know she had been placed in a full care facility, and did not realize that John was no longer at her side at all times. The terrible disease had erased all understanding from her brain, and had left just a very small part that was still Mary.

The skilled care facility that John and Ann chose was an excellent one and Mary received the best of care. John visited frequently, and so did Ann. Mary's condition continued to deteriorate, and almost three years later, she died.

Even though the disease totally destroyed Mary, John felt that he grew in his love for her through patience and understanding.

Ann felt fortunate to be able to share such an important task with her Dad, and this made daughter and father all the closer in their love for each other.

Ann and her husband also thought the experience had taught their children valuable lessons in caring, sharing and other important family values. They felt these lessons would help the children cope with life in an easier manner and with a better attitude.

Joe and Bob and their families never resented the fact that they spent vacations taking care of Mary instead of traveling. They felt it gave them a wonderful opportunity to function as a group and grow together in work and love.

Alzheimer's disease created a family tragedy for John, Mary, their children and grandchildren. Yet the illness also had unexpected positive effects, which will last for years to come.

Chapter Eleven
Conversations With Two Caregivers

I recommend you talk with other caregivers, people who are caring for their loved ones full time, in order to fully understand how it feels to deal with the disease all day, every day.

I remember, when my husband was ill, he was in and out of the hospital many times. Even though I was working full time, funds were low. I found myself running at breakneck speed daily. I am ashamed to admit that one day I asked myself, "What's in this for me?"

That's when I had to stop and have a long talk with myself. I had to decide where I was placing my values. I realized they were, of course, with the best interests of my sick husband. But sometimes we do have to stop and think about those things, and to look at how others have dealt with situations similar to ours.

I know two caregivers who were so loving of their patients and so open with their feelings, I felt their reactions would be valuable to others. On asking them to share their wisdom, they consented with open arms.

In the conversations that follow, I have once again changed names and circumstances to protect the privacy of others.

A conversation with Peggy

Peggy's mother had Alzheimer's disease over 20 years ago. Peggy is a registered nurse, and she and her siblings provided care for her mother. Her mother had the disease for 15 years, and was in a skilled care facility for eight years before she died.

Q: Peggy, you and I have been friends for so long. I wonder if you would share something very personal with me?

A: Sure, Eileen. What do you want me to share?

Q: I've been writing about Alzheimer's disease, trying to help caregivers understand the illness and its effects. I know your mother had Alzheimer's, and your family took care of her for many years. I wonder if you could give me some insight on how it feels to have a family member ill for such a long time?

A: I'd be glad to. I often reminisce about my mother. She worked hard bringing us up and she was good to all of us children, and to my children. If my thoughts can be of help to anyone, it will make me feel better, too.

Q: What were the first symptoms you noticed in your mother?

A: She would ask the same question over and over again. In the beginning it was occasional, but then became more frequent. Then she became acutely aware of her mistakes and our corrections. This caused her to become angry with us. I can remember her saying, "You're just trying to make me think I'm crazy." We would hug her and tell her, no, she had just made another mistake, and we loved her. She used to cry a lot and became depressed.

I remember another incident in the beginning of Mother's illness. Our family all had lunch together. About a half hour later I heard Mother in the kitchen. When I asked her what she was doing, she told me she was fixing lunch for us. She didn't even know she wasn't hungry. She had completely forgotten we had eaten.

That's when we were certain something was seriously wrong. I was so upset I just felt numb all over. I won't ever forget that feeling. We took Mother to the doctor and he confirmed our suspicions. He called it Chronic Brain Syndrome. What a cruel illness! I think there is a better understanding of Alzheimer's disease today than there was at that time.

Q: What was the progression of your mother's disease?

A: In the beginning she just made small errors or exercised poor judgment occasionally. That phase lasted about three years. Then we couldn't leave her alone any more. We worried about the stove, and other safety factors. She had also started wandering about the house and property aimlessly. Her play became inappropriate with the children. Several times she almost dropped the baby. Her speech was seriously affected, but she could still sing all the words to her favorite hymns and songs long after she had lost her speech. That phase lasted about three to four years.

She seemed to get worse as the day progressed. I've later heard it called "sundown syndrome." Before she died, we had totally reversed our roles. She fed me as a baby with a bottle. I fed Mother with a bottle before she died.

Q: Did you have any problems with friends and family staying away because of your mother's illness?

A: Not in any negative sense. They all were understanding and I spoke about Mother's illness freely. People reacted in many different ways to Mother's illness. My brother and his wife had a problem with it, and so did one of my sisters.

Q: What problem did your brother have?

A: My brother and his wife were wonderful, taking care of Mother. She lived with them after the early stages, and they cared for her with love until she needed to be placed in a skilled care facility for safety's sake. Our final decision not to keep Mother at home was determined in the middle of a cold winter night. We thought she was in bed. When we checked, we noticed she was gone. We found her in her nightgown, barefoot, down by the brook. My brother and his wife were so strong in caring for her, but neither could find it within themselves to place her. They felt like they were abandoning her.

My sister said, "I can't put my mother in one of those places. I can't take care of her all the time, either, because I have to work. I don't know what to do."

I told both of them, "You're off the hook. I know what needs to be done, and I will do it." Perhaps being a registered nurse allowed me to understand, and to have a different attitude. I knew I was doing the right thing. I loved Mother dearly, but her safety was at stake. She needed more protection than she could get at home.

My Dad was deceased for many years before Mother became ill. Our other siblings lived out of state and were not directly involved with her care. The whole problem came to rest on my shoulders. I knew what had to be done, and I did it.

Q: How did the rest of the family feel about you placing your mother in the facility?

A: They felt relieved, and their reactions and positive support made me feel I was glad I had the courage to do what I thought was right.

Q: What was the worst part of your mother's illness, for you?

A: Losing her before she died. She was always happy to see me when I went to visit her in the facility. She would smile and clap her hands. I think she thought I was just someone she liked. I don't think she knew I was her daughter. I think she thought I was a nice girl. I used to give her a big hug and say, "You're the best Mama in the whole wide world." She surprised me one day, long after she had stopped talking, by smiling a big smile and saying, "I know it." That made me wonder: How much does she really know? But that is something that will never be answered.

Q: Peggy, did your mother have much trouble adjusting to the skilled care facility?

A: I don't think she ever knew she was in different surroundings. In fact, I think the routine suited her better than the more flexible schedule at home.

I used to think it was a treat for her to bring her home on my day off. I'd bathe her and fix her hair and have her all to myself. Then I found out it took two or three days, after her visits, to get her back into a routine. She seemed to be over-stimulated when she returned. When they told me that, I didn't take her home with me any more. Instead, I visited frequently, even if it was for ten or fifteen minutes. I had to see that she was OK.

My brother and his wife visited her frequently, too. My sister visited occasionally. She would become so upset that she finally stopped visiting. She couldn't stand seeing her Mom that way. The grandchildren came by now and then and brought little goodies. The out-of-towners visited when they were near.

Q: Did the support group help you and your siblings?

A: I don't think there were any support groups for Alzheimer's disease in those days. We were a close family growing up and we have stayed close all these years. We supported each other.

A support group would have been a strong backing for us, to help us through the lonely time we all had to deal with during Mother's horrendous illness. Many times we all cried on each other's shoulders. We all learned that it's OK to cry. Then we would pick ourselves up, and smile, and do the work that was laid out before us. We were comforted by the fact that we had each other. We all had a wonderful mother. Knowing this gave us a positive outlook for the future.

Q: Peggy, what do you think was the hardest part of the illness for your mother?

A: The beginning of the illness was the worst. She was so aware of her errors and didn't know how to stop making mistakes. She thought she was crazy, that we didn't like her, and that we were making fun of her. She was so depressed and agitated. It hurt all of us to see her that way. I felt a great sense of relief when she became so ill that it seemed she didn't know anything. I truly hope she didn't know what was happening to her later on. She became docile and even seemed happy, although she was unable to speak.

Q: Do you have any advice for people faced with the problem of a loved one with Alzheimer's disease?

A: Just do what you can with a realistic viewpoint. There is no right time to keep the patient home or place them out of the home. Each person has to sit back and have their own personal decision time.

I think each person should be allowed to help or to visit according to his or her individual capacity. No one should be forced to care for or visit a sick person unless they feel good doing it. They should be excused. We all have a varied capacity for different things. Each person expresses their grief and caring in a personal way. That should be respected.

Contemplate what you are faced with and then design your plan objectively. You will have to do some things you would much prefer not to do, but then that's part of life. No one has a monopoly on the good or the bad.

A conversation with Sally

Sally's husband, Ed, is in Stage Five (Full Care) and has recently been placed in a skilled care facility.

Q: Sally, what was the first thing you noticed that warned you something was wrong with your husband?

A: I first noticed he was saying the wrong words for different things. For instance, I had my hair done at the beauty parlor and he greeted me by saying, "Oh, you got a new hat." Even though I noticed this, I didn't think too much about it.

Ed also did woodworking, and he was having trouble following the directions when it came to putting the things together. He made bookends that fit together the wrong way and put arms in the wrong place on wood figurines. I didn't realize anything was seriously wrong. I just figured he was getting older and he made mistakes. Then he stopped doing his woodworking altogether. I didn't think too much about that either.

Q: Who was the first person you told, when you thought something was wrong with Ed?

A: I didn't tell anyone. They told me. My son came for a visit from out of state after being away for about six months. He was shocked when he saw his father's behavior. He insisted we go to the doctor before he went back home.

Q: Do you think you really knew something was wrong with Ed all along, and just didn't want to believe it?

A: Yes. Now that I look back on it, I think I knew and foolishly was hoping it would go away. Maybe that's what they call denial.

Q: Do you think Ed knew something was wrong early in the disease?

A: Yes. I found one of his wood figurines in the trash and he never told me about having trouble making them, even after he stopped doing his woodworking. I also noticed his conversation was less and he was watching more and more TV. I think Ed knew he was using incorrect words and that he was having trouble in his conversation. Ed sort of became a little introverted.

Q: What was your initial reaction to Ed's illness when the doctor gave you the diagnosis?

A: I was totally devastated. I was frightened. I worried about my children getting the same illness. I didn't know what to do at first. But then as time went on and I learned more about Alzheimer's disease I developed a better perspective. I knew I would be able to cope with Ed's illness once I understood what I was dealing with, and knew what to expect in the future. He would have done the same for me if the situation had been reversed.

Q: Was there anything else you noticed early in the disease?

A: He experienced wide mood swings. Ed had always been a happy, peaceful man, and he would get depressed frequently but he didn't know why. Now that I under-stand the illness I can imagine what he was going through.

Q: What do you think was the most difficult part of the illness for Ed?

A: I think the gradual loss of words, thoughts and speech were so frustrating for him because he was aware of the loss. Sometimes he would try to tell me something and get so upset he would raise his hands and shake them and moan. I used to just hug him, then, and tell him how much I loved him, and sometimes he would cry quietly. It hurt me to see my big, strong man unable to do a simple thing like speaking.

Q: Did your children help you with their father's care?

A: They were wonderful. After the initial shock of their father's illness and they understood what was happening, they promised their help and all four of them kept their word. If things got too bad for me, one of them would come and stay with him and I would go to their house for a mini vacation. I don't think I could have done the care without their help. The grandchildren helped, too. He loved the kids and their play always made him happy. I think he felt he didn't have to prove himself with the little ones. He would truly relax with them.

Q: Did you ever use a skilled care facility for respite care for Ed?

A: Yes. We wanted to have a family reunion out of state. We knew it would be too much for Ed to handle. We also knew it would require constant watchfulness and care if we took Ed with us. We felt this was one time the family should feel free to relax together. We placed Ed in a facility that was recommended through our support group and the staff was wonderful. We all had a good time and came back feeling refreshed. Ed responded well to the trained staff at the facility.

Q: Do you think Ed still knows who you are?

A: I don't think he knows I'm his wife. I believe he thinks I'm someone who will help him all the time. He wants me with him all the time and that is impossible. Sometimes it seems like a little glimmer of the past shows in his eyes and then it's gone again.

Q: Do you think you lost some friends due to Ed's illness?

A: My good friends are still a wonderful support for me. Some acquaintances have not called since Ed became ill. I don't blame them. They just don't understand the illness and don't know what to say or do.

Q: Did any family stay away after Ed became ill?

A: One brother has stayed away. All the other members of the family have been a big help. I secretly feel that Ed's brother is afraid it will happen to him. He doesn't know what to say or do about it either. I've tried to help him understand the illness but he seems to listen with a closed mind. I hope one day he will come to see Ed again.

Q: Are you glad you decided to keep Ed home with you as long as possible?

A: Yes. It was very difficult, but on looking back on it, I wouldn't have had it any other way. I'm satisfied I did the best I could, and I did it with love. The work, the tears, the lost sleep have all been worth it.

Q: What was the most difficult part of taking care of Ed at home?

A: The constancy of it was the most difficult. Physically, it was wearing. Mentally, the worst part was watching him deteriorate and be less and less able to do things for himself. Sometimes I wished I could climb into his brain and pull out information. He would try to tell me something so hard yet couldn't verbalize his thoughts. I could feel his frustration mounting, and then he would stop trying to tell me whatever it was.

Q: What was the most difficult part of placing Ed in a skilled care facility?

A: I felt like I was abandoning him, even though I knew I wasn't. I was so tired and so frustrated, and I just prayed I had made the right decision. I miss him so much at home. I've also felt angry many times that we couldn't grow old gracefully together like so many other couples our age. Sometimes I feel jealous or resentful of them, and then I am ashamed of those feelings. But we had many good years together and I'm more than grateful for them. I visit him often and hold his hand, but I don't know how much of that he understands.

Q: Do you feel angry at life for doing this to you?

A: Yes, sometimes. I find myself wondering, "Why couldn't we get old together without all this trouble?" Yet on the other hand I'm glad I was well and able to help him through such a terrible ordeal for so long.

Q: Do you feel angry with Ed for getting sick?

A: No, not ever. He would have done the same for me if the situation had been reversed.

Q: Did the support group help you?

A: Tremendously. They were like a rock I could hold on to at the worst moments. I still go to the support group even though Ed is in a skilled care facility.

Q: Did day care help you?

A: It was wonderful. I could bring Ed there and know he was safe and well cared for while I relaxed from the constant care. It gave me time to gather myself together, either by going out with friends or going home to get some much needed rest.

Q: What haven't I asked that you would like to talk about?

A: Nothing in particular. There is one thought I have that I would like to share. We all have troubles of one sort or another. If we all put our troubles in one pile and then had to take one back, I think we would each take back our own. God is in charge, and after a while I think we all understand why we have the problems we do. That's my feeling, and you don't have to be any special religion to believe it. It helps me to think of it every day.

Postscript
ABOUT THE AUTHOR

During my high school years I always knew I wanted to help people. I decided at the time to become a registered nurse. Little did I know what a wonderful life, and what a feeling of fulfillment, that decision would give me.

I was a registered nurse for 44 years, then retired in 1989. I soon became restless, and for three years prior to writing this book, I worked part time at an Alzheimer's day care facility.

I started nurses' training in 1944 and have worked since then in the medical field, with few interruptions. I attended a three-year diploma school with the Franciscan Sisters of the Sick Poor in New York City. The Sisters were strict and hard task masters. Many times since graduation I have said a silent thank-you to them for the lessons I learned. I may have resented their strictness when in school, but appreciated it later in difficult situations.

My first job after graduation was in a hospital operating room. How fascinating was the work the doctors were able to do! Yet I missed the flow of patients, and left after two years.

I next worked with a dedicated general practitioner in Brooklyn in the late '40s. During this time, we had the advent of antibiotics, many wonderful machines, tranquilizers and other medical miracles we take very much for granted today. The doctor had such a wonderful attitude toward his patients, it was not a job but a pleasure being his assistant. (I regret to say he died in 1992 of Alzheimer's disease, at the age of 86.) It was with him I first experienced working with entire families for extended periods of time.

Things were different back in those days. If a patient was sick, either in or out of the hospital, and couldn't find a nurse, guess who the doctor would call? That's right: me. I'd always go. After the crisis was over, it was such a reward to have someone well again that all the work was worth the trouble. When the doctor delivered babies we often knew all the aunts, uncles, cousins and sometimes the neighbors. This experience gave me an inside look at how one person's medical condition can affect an entire family.

I left the doctor after 12 years to help my husband in business. Once again I missed the flow of patients. Before long I decided to work one or two days a week in a hospital. Pretty soon I was working full time again and my husband had hired other help. I found the hospital to be a source of instant rewards, 100 times a day. That was where I belonged.

Time went by and a former patient came to visit me. He was the manager of a large industrial building in metropolitan New York, and he wanted to open an emergency medical unit for the employees. He invited me to be in charge of it. What a challenge! I felt rather nervous because I would be the only medical personnel available for emergencies. I went back to the dear doctor I had spent so much time with and told him about the offer. He assured me I could do it and said, "Just exercise good judgment." I took the job, and once again I was able to get to know the same people over an extended period of time.

In 1977 I moved to Florida. My husband had retired with a disability, and the New York winters were difficult for him. I worked at another hospital, full time. We had more elderly people in our cross section of patients than there were up north. Many had Alzheimer's disease.

Medical care was beginning to change, becoming more impersonal. I thought it would be good to do some home nursing and really get to know the families. When you do nursing in the home you become part of the family's daily life. I saw six to eight patients on a regular basis. Many of these people were dealing with Alzheimer's disease.

From there I went to work at a retirement home. It was an ideal place for elderly people to live. We had the people divided into four categories: Well (they signed in and out at will); Partial Care (they needed some help bathing or dressing, due to Alzheimer's disease and other disabilities); Full Care (needed help with all activities of daily living, due to various illnesses); Infirmary (people with acute illnesses who required intensive nursing care). With such a large group of elderly people under one roof we had many with Alzheimer's disease. They were all well cared for.

When I reached age 62 I retired. I felt I was slowing down and the pace was too fast for me. I declared I was no longer a nurse. Yet I was bored staying home all the time and needed more activity. A job in one of the better department stores was my next endeavor. That didn't work. I didn't fit, and I left. What, I wondered, should I do next? I had allowed my nursing license to expire in March of '91.

How lucky I was: An Alzheimer's day care center hired me as a part time activity assistant. Once again I was involved with families. I saw that they all shared a big problem, and many had no idea how to cope. I decided to put into writing some of the things I had seen and done.

We all gather information as we go through life. It feels good to put that information down on paper in an effort to help others.

Since I am a rather restless creature, moving from state to state, I have been exposed to many varied situations. I was never sorry about my career choice. Nursing gives you a feeling daily of having done some good for your fellow man. We all get a chance to pattern our lives, and I have been content with mine.

No more to tell about me.

Eileen Higgins Driscoll
R.N.(retired)

REFERENCES

Alzheimers Association
919 North Michigan Avenue
Suite 1000
Chicago, Illinois 60611-1676
Phone: (312) 335-9602
Fax: (312) 335-0214

Department of Health and Human Services
6325 Security Boulevard
Baltimore,Maryland 21207
Social Security
Phone: 1-800-772-1213
Medicare Hot-line
1-800-638-6833
Low Low Income Benefits

AARP/ American Association of Retired People
601 E Street NW
Washington DC, 20049
1-800-424-3410
(They offer an excellent booklet
Coping & Caring Living With Alzheimer's disease

Alzheimer's disease Education and Referal Center
P.O.Box 8250
Silver Springs, Maryland 20907-8250
1-800-438-4380
General Information Packet

American Health Assistance Foundation
Alzheimer's Family Relief Program
Educational Materials
Manager: Joyce Thelen
Financial assistance if qualified.
15825 Shady Grove Road
Suite 140
Rockville,Maryland 20850
1 800 437 2423

National Hospice Organization
1901 North Moore Street
Suite 901
Arlington, Virginia 22209
703 243 5900
800 658 8898

Department of Health and Human Services
Administration on Aging (AOA)
Assistant Secretary for Aging:
Dr. Fernando Torres-Gil, Ph.D.
330 Independence Avenue SW
Room 4760
Washington, D.C. 20201
202-401-4634

Meals-on-Wheels national office.
Your local Alzheimer's Association can give you the telephone number in your area. They do not serve all areas in the country.

National Association of Area Agencies on Aging
1112 16th Street NW
Suite 100
Washington, D.C. 20036
202-296-8130

Transportation   No national office
Your local Alzheimer's Association can advise you on transportation available in your area at a reduced cost if it is available.

Home Health Aid will come through your personal physician or local Alzheimer's Association if available.

Related Reading Material

Alzheimer's disease
A Practical Guide for Families and Other Caregivers
Judah L. Ronch

Alzheimer's
Caring For Your Loved One
Caring For Yourself
Sharon Fish

Alzheimer's disease
William A. Check

When Your Loved One Has Alzheimer's
David L. Carroll

Facing Alzheimer's
Patricia Brown Coughlan

The Loss of Self
Donna Cohen,Ph. D.
Carl Eisdorfer, Ph. D.,M.D.

The 36 Hour Day
Nancy Mace and Peter V. Rabins M.D.

Caring For Alzheimer's Patients
Gary D. Miner, Ph.D.
Linda A. Winters-Miner, Ph.D.
John P. Blass, M.D. Ph.D.
Ralph W. Richter, M.D.
Jimmie L. Valentine, Ph.D.

Related Videos for viewing

Your local Public Library should have copies of these videos.

Alzheimer's disease /Scripps Clinic Health Report

Just For The Summer...This is an excellent tool to help children understand Alzheimer's disease.

There Were Times Dear

Sundown: Coping With Alzheimer's

Alzheimers: Effects on Patients and Their Families

BOOKS ON HEALTH-RELATED ISSUES

AIDS READER--Documentary History of a Modern Epidemic by Loren Clark and Malcolm Potts is an anthology on the history and impact of AIDS by some of the world's great experts. Paper, ISBN 0-8283-1918-9, $17.95.

ALZHEIMER'S--A Handbook for the Caretaker by Eileen Driscoll, a nurse with several decades f experience, gives hope to those having to cope with alzheimer patients. Paper, ISBN 0-8283-1962-6, $12.95.

AUTISM--From Tragedy to Triumph by Carol Johnson and Julia Crowder--the mother--tells the story of a young man, from birth to college matriculation. Paper, ill., ISBN 0-8283-1965-0, $12.95.

HINDU PSYCHOLOGY--Meaning for the West by Akhilananda explores, in clear style, the impact of Hinduism on the West. Paper, ISBN 0-8283-1353-9, $14.95.

MAKING WISE CHOICES--A Guide for Women by Charlotte Thompson, M.D. contains a series of essays on crucial issues confronting women--married or single, especially those who may have to make it alone. Paper, ISBN 0-8283-1972-3, $12.95.

MARIJUANA--Up-Date by Dr. Richard Robbins presents extensive research done by civilian and military personnel on the use and abuse of this drug. Paper, ISBN 0-8283-1856-5, $11.95.

MENTAL HEALTH AND HINDU PSYCHOLOGY by Akhilananda has become a classic in this field. Paper, ISBN 0-8283-1354-7, $14.95.

PARKINSON'S--A Personal Story of Acceptance by Sandi Gordon is the autobiography of Sandi as a woman, a mother and patient suffering from this dreadful and common disease. Illustrated. 1949-9 $12.95 p.

PUMPKIN--A Young Woman's Struggle with Lupus by Patricia Fagan--the mother and professional nurse--tells the story of 'Pumpkin', and her relationship with relatives and friends. Paper, ISBN 0-8283-1961-8, $12.95.

**Entire text was produced with *Pages and Windows*
for WordPerfect 5.1 (DOS)**